Case Compendium in ENDOCRINOLOGY

Case Compendium in ENDOCRINOLOGY

Editor

Romesh Khardori MD PhD FRCP(C) FACP
Professor of Medicine
Division of Endocrinology and Metabolism
Strelitz Center for Diabetes, Endocrine, and Metabolic Disorders
Department of Internal Medicine
Eastern Virginia Medical School
Norfolk, Virginia, USA

Associate Editors

Sarita Bajaj MD DM
Consultant Endocrinologist
Director-Professor and Head
Department of Medicine
Moti Lal Nehru Medical College
Allahabad, Uttar Pradesh, India

Smita Gupta MD
Consultant Endocrinologist
Community Health Network
Indianapolis, Indiana, USA

JAYPEE *The Health Sciences Publisher*

New Delhi | London | Philadelphia | Panama

Jaypee Brothers Medical Publishers (P) Ltd

Headquarters

Jaypee Brothers Medical Publishers (P) Ltd
4838/24, Ansari Road, Daryaganj
New Delhi 110 002, India
Phone: +91-11-43574357
Fax: +91-11-43574314
Email: jaypee@jaypeebrothers.com

Overseas Offices

J.P. Medical Ltd
83 Victoria Street, London
SW1H 0HW (UK)
Phone: +44 20 3170 8910
Fax: +44 (0)20 3008 6180
Email: info@jpmedpub.com

Jaypee-Highlights Medical Publishers Inc
City of Knowledge, Bld. 237, Clayton
Panama City, Panama
Phone: +1 507-301-0496
Fax: +1 507-301-0499
Email: cservice@jphmedical.com

Jaypee Medical Inc
The Bourse
111 South Independence Mall East
Suite 835, Philadelphia, PA 19106, USA
Phone: +1 267-519-9789
Email: jpmed.us@gmail.com

Jaypee Brothers Medical Publishers (P) Ltd
17/1-B Babar Road, Block-B, Shaymali
Mohammadpur, Dhaka-1207
Bangladesh
Mobile: +08801912003485
Email: jaypeedhaka@gmail.com

Jaypee Brothers Medical Publishers (P) Ltd
Bhotahity, Kathmandu, Nepal
Phone: +977-9741283608
Email: kathmandu@jaypeebrothers.com

Website: www.jaypeebrothers.com
Website: www.jaypeedigital.com

Inquiries for bulk sales may be solicited at: jaypee@jaypeebrothers.com

Case Compendium in Endocrinology

First Edition: **2015**

ISBN: 978-93-5152-643-8

Printed at: Ajanta Offset & Packagings Ltd., New Delhi

Dedicated to

Pursuit of excellence in quest of acquisition of knowledge and delivery of care to patients whose interests reign supreme

Contents

Contributors

EDITOR

Romesh Khardori MD PhD FRCP(C) FACP
Professor of Medicine
Division of Endocrinology and Metabolism
Strelitz Center for Diabetes, Endocrine, and Metabolic Disorders
Department of Internal Medicine
Eastern Virginia Medical School
Norfolk, Virginia, USA

ASSOCIATE EDITORS

Sarita Bajaj MD DM
Consultant Endocrinologist
Director-Professor and Head
Department of Medicine
Moti Lal Nehru Medical College
Allahabad, Uttar Pradesh, India

Smita Gupta MD
Consultant Endocrinologist
Community Health Network
Indianapolis, Indiana, USA

CONTRIBUTING AUTHORS

Mini R Abraham MD
Consultant Endocrinologist
Overland Park Medical Specialists
Overland Park, Kansa, USA

Joseph A Aloi MD FACP FACE
Professor and Section Chief
Division of Endocrinology
Wake Forest University School of Medicine
Winston, North Carolina, USA

AC Ammini MD DM
Professor and Head
Department of Endocrinology
All India Institute of Medical Sciences
New Delhi, India

Manjunath G Anakal MD DM
Assistant Professor
Department of Medicine
MR Medical College
Gulbarga, Karnataka, India

Vageesh Ayyar S MD DM DNB MNAMS
Additional Professor
Department of Endocrinology
St John's Medical College and Hospital
Bengaluru, Karnataka, India

Naresh Bansal MD
Senior Resident
Department of Endocrinology and Metabolism
Institute of Medical Sciences
Varanasi, Uttar Pradesh, India

Ganapathi Bantwal MD DM DNB MNAMS
Professor and Head
Department of Endocrinology
St John's Medical College and Hospital
Bengaluru, Karnataka, India

Mir Iftikhar Bashir MD DM
Additional Professor
Sher-e-Kashmir Institute of Medical Sciences
Srinagar, Jammu and Kashmir, India

Vijayalakshmi Bhatia MBBS MD
Professor
Department of Endocrinology
Sanjay Gandhi Postgraduate Institute of Medical Sciences
Lucknow, Uttar Pradesh, India

Eesh Bhatia MD DNB
Professor and Head
Department of Endocrinology
Sanjay Gandhi Postgraduate Institute of Medical Sciences
Lucknow, Uttar Pradesh, India

Vijaykumar S Bhavi MBBS MD
Assistant Professor
Department of Medicine
SDM Medical College
Dharwad, Karnataka, India

Danielle OM Castillo MD
Division of Endocrinology and Metabolism
Eastern Virginia Medical School
Norfolk, Virginia, USA

Akshat Chadha MBBS MBA
Consultant Physician
Hope and Care Center
Mumbai, Maharashtra, India

Manoj Chadha MD DM
Consultant Endocrinologist
PD Hinduja Hospital and Research Centre
Mumbai, Maharashtra, India

Celine Chaya MD
Fellow in Endocrinology
Department of Endocrinology
Eastern Virginia Medical School
Norfolk, Virginia, USA

Mala Dharmalingam DM
Professor
Department of Endocrinology
MS Ramaiah Medical College
Bengaluru, Karnataka, India

Vinay Dipali MD DM
Senior Resident
Department of Endocrinology
St John's Medical College and Hospital
Bengaluru, Karnataka, India

Belinda George MD DM
Assistant Professor
Department of Endocrinology
St John's Medical College and Hospital
Bengaluru, Karnataka, India

Vasudha Goel MD
Senior Resident
Department of Medicine
Pandit Bhagwat Dayal Sharma Post Graduate Institute of Medical Sciences
Rohtak, Haryana, India

Ketan G Goswami MD FACE
Consultant Endocrinologist
Gwinnett Medical Center
Lawrenceville, Georgia, USA

Sridhar R Gumpeny MD DM FACE FRCP
Director
Endocrine and Diabetes Center
Visakhapatnam, Andhra Pradesh, India

RV Jayakumar MD DM MNAMS FRCP
Professor
Department of Endocrinology
Amrita Institute of Medical Sciences
School of Medicine
Kochi, Kerala, India

Parjeet Kaur MD DM
Consultant
Department of Endocrinology and Diabetes
Medanta, The Medicity
Gurgaon, Haryana, India

Narendra Kotwal MD DNB DM
Professor
Department of Endocrinology
Army Hospital R&R
New Delhi, India

KM Prasanna Kumar MD DM
Consultant Endocrinologist
Bangalore Diabetes Hospital—CDEC
Bengaluru, Karnataka, India

David C Lieb MD
Associate Professor
Division of Endocrinology
Department of Medicine
Program Director, Endocrinology and Metabolism Fellowship Program
Eastern Virginia Medical School
Norfolk, Virginia, USA

Debashish Maji MD DM
Professor and Head
Department of Medicine
Vivekananda Institute of Medical Sciences
Kolkata, West Bengal, India

Sunil K Mishra MD DM
Senior Consultant
Department of Endocrinology and Diabetes, Medanta, The Medicity
Gurgaon, Haryana, India

Ambrish Mithal MD DM
Chairman
Department of Endocrinology and Diabetes, Medanta, The Medicity
Gurgaon, Haryana, India

John T O'Brian MD FACP
Professor of Medicine
Division of Endocrinology and Metabolism
Eastern Virginia Medical School
Norfolk, Virginia, USA

Girish Parmar DNB (Medicine) DNB (Endo)
Consultant Endocrinologist
KD Ambani Hospital
Mumbai, Maharashtra, India

Rajesh Rajput MD DM FICP FIACM FIMSA
Senior Professor and Head
Department of Medicine and Endocrinology
Pandit Bhagwat Dayal Sharma Post Graduate Institute of Medical Sciences
Rohtak, Haryana, India

Mandip S Rawla MBBS ABIM
Fellow
Division of Endocrinology and Metabolism
Eastern Virginia Medical School
Norfolk, Virginia, USA

Donald W Richardson BA MD AOA
Associate Professor
Department of Endocrinology and Metabolism
Eastern Virginia Medical School
Norfolk, Virginia, USA

Narasimha KR Setty MD
Director
Karnataka Institute of Diabetology
Bengaluru, Karnataka, India

Shruti Sharma MD DM
Senior Resident
Department of Endocrinology and Metabolism
Institute of Medical Sciences
Varanasi, Uttar Pradesh, India

Surekha B Shetty MD
Consultant Diabetologist
Karnataka Institute of Diabetology
Bengaluru, Karnataka, India

Surya K Singh MD DM
Professor
Department of Endocrinology and Metabolism
Institute of Medical Sciences
Banaras Hindu University
Varanasi, Uttar Pradesh, India

Siddnath Sudhanshu MBBS MD PDCC
Fellow Resident
Department of Endocrinology
Sanjay Gandhi Postgraduate Institute of Medical Sciences
Lucknow, Uttar Pradesh, India

Jagdeesh Ullal MD MS CCD ECNU FACE FACP
Assistant Professor
Division of Endocrinology and Metabolism
Eastern Virginia Medical School
Norfolk, Virginia, USA

Lauren A Willard DO
Assistant Professor
Department of Medicine
Division of Endocrinology
University of Pittsburgh Medical Centre
Pittsburgh, Pennsylvania, USA

Abdul H Zargar MD DM
Professor
Department of Endocrinology
Sher-e-Kashmir Institute of Medical Sciences
Srinagar, Jammu and Kashmir, India

Preface

Any attempt to format a book designed to convey essence of inquiry into pathologic states experienced by patients, must be rooted in desire on part of learners to understand fundamentals of physiologic principles governing the system under investigation. That knowledge must be gained by rigorous study of physiology from reliable sources. Cliff notes and self-study guides do not convey the art and the beauty of studying details that only standard reference textbooks provide. While writing and editing cases for the "Case Compendium", we charged the authors with describing an interesting case and building discussion around the case in a manner that would allow a learner to think through a case like a detective who is sifting through data from crime scene and constructing a story that helps solve the mystery. We did not go into details of physiology, as a learner pursuing specialization in endocrinology would have taken upon himself/herself to study physiology and contemporary biology as a prerequisite to pursue higher studies. It is with this background that we have asked our authors to contribute their thoughts and images which was crucial to our planning of every chapter. Their inputs make this compendium possible.

We have attempted to provide a case history along with relevant data from physical examination and investigative studies. Differential diagnosis has been constructed around case under study, and the reader is then guided through discussion that helps explain the case. This approach is a departure from many similar books where differential diagnosis is often not focused upon and rather than addressing the patient under discussion, differential diagnosis focusses on the disease entity in particular. We believe a focused differential diagnosis simulates a real life situation better, and prepares reader to think while on their toes.

We have also provided a short list of suggested readings worthy of reading at the end of each case. This list is deliberately kept short to avoid pitfall of turning a case discussion into an exhaustive review that could be distracting. The compendium is a mixture of routine and some very interesting cases. It is our hope that learners will find the format easy to navigate and at the same time loaded with information that is relevant and highly pertinent. We hope that we are provided feedback to help us design the next volume.

Romesh Khardori
Sarita Bajaj
Smita Gupta

Acknowledgments

Editors wish to acknowledge the unconditional support of Dr Neeraj Choudhary, Senior Editor, in engaging the Editors and Authors in compilation of this work. The publisher has been gracious in offering support without any interference whatsoever, and the team has also ensured that the quality of work is superb.

This compendium would not have seen the light of the day without untiring effort of Ms Shweta Tiwari, Editorial Coordinator, who provided oversight on behalf of publishers.

Finally, we wish to acknowledge our debt of gratitude to all contributing authors, who were patient with our requests and edits.

CHAPTER

1

Primary Ovarian Insufficiency

Girish Parmar, Akshata Chadha, Manoj Chadha

CASE PRESENTATION

A 26-year-old female presented with a history of amenorrhea for last 6 months. She had undergone normal puberty with menarche at 12 years of age. Her menses were regular for the next 10 years but subsequently became irregular. She had oligomenorrhea and once had no menses for 6 months. She started taking oral contraceptive pills (OCP) for irregular menses since the last 2 years to which she had regular withdrawal bleed. She had gone off OCP for last 6 months when seen at endocrine clinic. Her weight is 59 kg and her height 166 cm. Her body mass index is 21.3 kg/m^2 and waist circumference of 79 cm. There is no acanthosis, goiter, galactorrhea, hirsutism, or acne. There is no easy bruising, proximal muscle weakness, or livid purple striae. The pelvic examination is normal, a pregnancy test is negative, thyroid-stimulating hormone level is 2.67 mIU/L, prolactin level is 12 ng/mL (normal: <23 ng/mL), and follicle-stimulating hormone is 68 IU/L (in the menopausal range). How should she be evaluated and treated?

PERTINENT INVESTIGATIONS FOR EVALUATING A CASE OF AMENORRHEA

- Follicle-stimulating hormone (FSH), luteinizing hormone
- Estradiol
- Ultrasonography pelvis for status of ovaries (follicles) and outflow tract
- Thyroid-stimulating hormone (TSH), prolactin.

DIFFERENTIAL DIAGNOSIS

Based on the clinical features, the differential diagnosis would revolve around:

- Pregnancy
- Hypothalamic amenorrhea (chronic emotional stress, malnutrition, anorexia)
- Weight loss (nutritional deprivation/malnutrition)
- Thyroid dysfunction
- Hyperprolactinemia
- Polycystic ovary syndrome
- Primary ovarian insufficiency
- Congenital adrenal hyperplasia/hyperandrogenemia
- Pituitary insufficiency (destruction—tumors, infiltration, and hypophysitis)
- Hypersecretory pituitary disorders (Cushing's disease, acromegaly).

In this particular case, several potential conditions can be excluded based on the data provided (nonpregnant, normal TSH, and prolactin with elevated FSH level). These include pregnancy, polycystic ovary syndrome (PCOS), hyperprolactinemia, hyperandrogenemia, hypopituitarism, pituitary hypersecretory disorders, hypothalamic amenorrhea, and thyroid dysfunction. The differential diagnosis is rather limited. In none of the conditions enumerated above would the FSH level be elevated. An elevated FSH level (confirmed on repeat testing) indicates ovarian insufficiency. Therefore, primary concern should be about primary ovarian insufficiency (POI).

Based on the clinical features and the laboratory details, the differential diagnosis is narrowed to:

- Primary ovarian insufficiency (syndromic, nonsyndromic gene mutations)
- Autoimmune/toxic oophoritis
- Pituitary tumor (FSH secreting)
- Inactivating mutation of follicle-stimulating hormone receptor (primary amenorrhea most common).

DISCUSSION

Activation of the hypothalamo-pituitary-gonadal (HPG) axis at the time of puberty leads to gradual emergence of secondary sexual characters culminating in menstruation and leading to achievement of reproductive capability. At puberty menses are usually irregular and may remain so in 20–30% of adolescents for a period of 3 years from menarche. Subsequently, menses become predictable at regular intervals. The vignette case had experienced puberty that was normal in timing and development, indicating normal functioning of HPG axis at that point of time. It also indicates presence of an intact uterus and outflow tract. Subsequently, menses were regular for a decade until it became irregular. Irregular menses is an indication of anovulation.

The fact the FSH levels are in menopausal range indicates ovarian failure/insufficiency. Primary ovarian insufficiency is the preferred term for this condition, as was originally coined by Fuller Albright in 1942. It signifies that this disorder is not irretrievably irreversible. Earlier term like premature menopause has been inappropriately used. This term is inaccurate since 5–10% of women conceive and deliver even after the diagnosis. Moreover, menopause denotes depletion of functional primordial follicles resulting in permanent cessation of menses. Menopause before the age of 40 years has been defined as premature. Terms like hypergonadotropic amenorrhea, hypergonadotropic hypogonadism, primary hypogonadism, resistant ovary, or Savage syndrome are no longer used.

Primary ovarian insufficiency should be considered when a woman <40 years of age has had amenorrhea/disordered menses for at least 4 months or more, with two serum FSH levels in the menopausal range (separated by one month interval). There is no established cutoff for FSH concentration to suggest ovarian insufficiency due to erratic and intermittent decline ovarian function.

The age-specific incidence of 46XX spontaneous POI is approximately 1 in 250 by age 35 years, and 1 in 100 by age 40 years. In 90% of the cases, etiology of POI remains unclear. Spontaneous 46XX POI can occasionally occur as part of a defined phenotype/syndrome or as a consequence of single gene mutations. Several candidate genes have been identified of which most significant ones are *FMR1, AIRE, STAR GALT, ATM, BLM*, and *WRN*.

Primary ovarian insufficiency arises from either dysfunctional gonadotropin–ovarian interaction (mutation in FSH receptor), and mutations involving postreceptor steps in FSH action, or depletion of ovarian primordial follicles. Etiology in majority of POI cases is often not determined; however, X chromosome abnormalities (13%), autoimmunity (4–30%), and fragile X premutations (6%) predominate. Thus, karyotyping and testing for *FMR1* mutation, testing for adrenal, and thyroid antibodies would be in order. Pelvic ultrasound to look for ovarian morphology is recommended, while testing for ovarian antibody or ovarian biopsy is not recommended.

CLINICAL FEATURES

Symptoms of estrogen deficiency such as hot flashes, night sweats, sleep disturbance, and dyspareunia (secondary to vaginal dryness) are common in most patients with POI. Osteopenia and osteoporosis are common in young women who develop ovarian dysfunction before they achieve peak adult bone mass. Impaired endothelial function, increased cardiovascular morbidity and mortality, possibly related to endothelial dysfunction are seen in patients undergoing bilateral oophorectomy before age 45 years.

A positive family history, with an affected first-degree relative, may be found in approximately 10–15% of cases. This would strongly favor search for autoimmune disorders such as hypothyroidism, adrenal insufficiency, and hypoparathyroidism. A positive family history for fragile X syndrome points to a permutation in *FMR1* gene. This permutation is the second most common cause of primary ovarian failure after Turner's syndrome. Other familial disorders of interest include mutations of *ATM, FOXL2,* and *GALT* associated, respectively, with ataxia telangiectasia, blepharophimosis-ptosis-epicanthus-inversus syndrome, and galactosemia.

Physical examination may provide vital clues of an associated disorder such as thyromegaly, vitiligo, dry eye, short digits, short stature, and lack of breast development.

MANAGEMENT

Regardless of the known intermittency of ovarian function, women with POI should receive estrogen therapy to prevent bone loss, hot flashes, night sweats, dyspareunia, and cognitive impairment (with a progestin to protect against endometrial cancer). In addition to estrogen, other important measures for bone health should be emphasized, including exercise, adequate calcium and vitamin D intake, and avoiding smoking. The current approach is to treat with a hormone replacement regimen that mimics normal physiology as closely as possible until the average age of natural menopause. Type of estrogen therapy and optimal replacement with sex steroids depends on individual needs. Girls or young women with primary amenorrhea in whom secondary sex characteristics have failed to develop should initially be given very low doses of estrogen (at first without a progestin) in an attempt to mimic gradual pubertal maturation.

The principal estrogen produced by the functioning premenopausal ovary is 17β-estradiol. Hormone replacement for young women with POI should mimic normal ovarian function as much as possible. To control vasomotor symptoms and to fully estrogenize the vaginal epithelium, most women with spontaneous POI are started on full replacement doses of estrogen such as transdermal estradiol (usually 100 μg daily) or oral estradiol (usually 2 mg/day). This usually achieves circulating E2 levels of approximately 100 pg/mL (typical average found in during normal menstrual cycle).

Alternatively, conjugated estrogen in doses of 0.625–1.25 mg may be used. In patients with intact uterus, medroxyprogesterone acetate (5–10 mg) or micronized progesterone (100–200 mg) may be given for 14 days every 30–60 days. This is done to avoid estrogen induced endometrial hyperplasia. Patients should experience withdrawal bleed, and failure to do so should prompt a pregnancy test.

Providing estradiol by transdermal patch has several advantages:

- It provides 17β-estradiol, which is structurally identical to ovarian 17β-estradiol
- It avoids the first pass effect on the liver
- It provides the replacement by steady infusion rather than by bolus
- It reduces the risk of venous thromboembolism compared with the oral route and may be associated with a reduced risk of gallbladder disease (i.e. cholecystitis and cholelithiasis).

Since spontaneous ovarian activity may resume, some form of contraception may be warranted if pregnancy is not desired. It is uncertain whether administration of physiologic doses of estrogen followed sequentially by a progestin is better for skeletal health than pharmacologic doses of a combined estrogen-progestin regimen (i.e. oral contraceptives). Adequate daily intake of calcium and vitamin D is recommended. Bisphosphonates are avoided if pregnancy is possible since effects on developing fetus are unknown.

In ultrasonographic studies of women with POI, follicular development occurs frequently, but ovulation is infrequent, with evidence of luteinization in many cases. However, exogenous administration of physiologic doses of estrogen does not appear to improve the spontaneous ovulation rate. This was shown in a trial of 37 women with POI randomly assigned to receive oral estradiol (2 mg/day) or no therapy for 6 weeks in a 12-week crossover design. No effect of oral estradiol replacement was seen on mean ovarian volume, the number or size of new follicles, or ovulatory rates. Given the small size of this study, a possible benefit of estrogen cannot be excluded.

There are no established, prospectively proven safe and effective treatments that will restore ovulation in women with POI. Ovulation induction with gonadotropin therapy is often attempted, but ovulation and pregnancy rates are low. Exogenous gonadotropins could theoretically exacerbate unrecognized autoimmune ovarian failure. Suppression of endogenous gonadotropin concentrations with pharmacologic doses of estrogen prior to gonadotropin therapy has been reported to improve ovulatory rates in some, but not all studies. In one randomized placebo-controlled trial, treatment with 150 μg ethinyl estradiol/day for 2 weeks before and during stimulation with recombinant FSH, ovulatory rates were significantly higher in the estrogen group (32%; 8 of 25 women) when compared with the placebo group (0 of 25 ovulated). Ovulation only occurred in women whose serum FSH concentrations were suppressed to ≤15 IU/L with estrogen.

Women with POI due to any cause are potential candidates for in vitro fertilization with donor oocytes. Success rates for this procedure depend primarily on the age of the oocyte donor.

As with any life-altering diagnosis, women with POI benefit from encouragement and support that helps them to regain a sense of control and confidence. Studies reveal that women with POI have more complaints of anxiety, depression, low self-esteem, and lower satisfaction with their sex lives.

KEY POINTS

- Primary ovarian insufficiency is not a rare disorder in clinical practice and spans across a spectrum of menstrual disorders and not just amenorrhea only
- Early diagnosis necessary for initiation of appropriate hormone replacement
- Hormone replacement therapy should be continued till average age of menopause
- Primary ovarian insufficiency may reverse spontaneously or on treatment with estrogen.

SUGGESTED READINGS

1. De Vos M, Devroey P, Fauser CJM. Primary ovarian insufficiency. Lancet. 2010;310:911-92.
2. Doherty E, Pakarinen P, Tiitinen A, et al. A novel mutation in FSH receptor inhibiting signal transduction and causing premature ovarian failure. J Clin Endocrinol Metab. 2002;87:1151-5.
3. Hawkins S, Matzuk M. The menstrual cycle basic biology. Ann NY Acad Sci. 2008;1135:10-8.
4. Nelson LM. Clinical practice: primary ovarian insufficiency. N Engl J Med. 2009;360:606-14.
5. Roberts-Wilson TK, Spencer JB, Frantz C. Using an algorithmic approach to secondary amenorrhea. Clinica Chemica Acta. 2013;423:56-61.
6. Tuohy V, Altuntas C. Autoimmunity and premature ovarian failure. Cur Opin Obstet Gynecol. 2007; 19:366-9.

CHAPTER

2

Subacute Thyroiditis

Mala Dharmalingam, Manjunath G Anakal

CASE PRESENTATION

A 24-year-old lady Ms G first presented in July 2010 with complaints of pain in front of the neck radiating to left upper jaw associated with mild fever, body ache, and palpitations for preceding 15 days. She was seen by a dentist and treated symptomatically for pain and fever. Two-weeks later she developed pain on the right side of neck, associated with increasing tiredness. She was suspected to have hyperthyroidism and referred to endocrinologist. During interview, she reported tremors, sweating, and weight loss for the last 2 months. On physical examination, her pulse rate was 120 beats/minute (high volume and regular rhythm); blood pressure was 150/70 mmHg; and she was pale. There was no pedal edema or jaundice. On palpation of the thyroid gland it was diffusely enlarged, and the margins were well defined and it was tender on examination. There was no bruit on auscultation. Systemic examination was unremarkable.

LABORATORY/IMAGING EVALUATION

- Thyroid stimulating hormone (TSH): 0.005 μIU/mL (normal: 0.25–5 μIU/mL)
- Total T4: >22 μg/dL (normal: 4.5–12 μg/dL)
- T3: 250 ng/dL (normal: 80–230 ng/dL)
- Thyroid peroxidase (TPO) antibodies: 138.9 μIU/mL (normal: <35 μIU/mL)
- High thyroglobulin levels >1,300 ng/mL (normal: 2–35 ng/mL)
- Erythrocyte sedimentation rate (ESR): 40 mm in first hour
- Complete blood count: Normal
- Thyroid-ultrasonography: Hypoechogenicity of right lobe and normal echotexture of the left lobe
- Technetium-99 scan: There was no uptake in the thyroid region consistent with thyroiditis.

She was treated symptomatically and reassured. She revisited after 2 months with persistent symptoms of hyperthyroidism. She was once again reassured and asked to come after 1 month. She came back a month later with symptoms of hypothyroidism, severe muscle cramps and myalgia with a weight gain of 3 kg. On further evaluation, TSH level was >100 μIU/mL. She was placed on levothyroxine replacement. She came back after 2 months, with symptoms of hyperthyroidism. At this time, TSH level was <0.001 μIU/mL and total T4 level was 18 μg/dL. On the assumption that it was iatrogenic hyperthyroidism, levothyroxine was stopped. She was reassured and asked to come back after 2 months. She came back after 2 months with toxic symptoms and biochemically hyperthyroid. A diagnosis of recurrent thyroiditis was made, she was again treated symptomatically with β-blockers; on follow-up after 6 months, TSH level was 14 μIU/mL and T4 was 3 μg/dL. Since she was asymptomatic, no treatment was started. However, 2 months later she came with severe hyperthyroid symptoms and thyroid function tests in the hyperthyroid range. This time she was given a course of analgesics for symptomatic improvement. She improved when she was on steroids; however after 3 months when the steroid was tapered off she again became hyperthyroid. In the process, she had both technetium scan and also a radioiodine scan. Both of which showed a poor uptake. Though recurrent subacute thyroiditis (SAT) is very rare (4%), our patient fits this diagnosis. A decision to recommend thyroidectomy was made. She underwent total thyroidectomy in June 2012. She became hypothyroid and was started on thyroxin replacement. She is now doing fine on follow-up.

DIFFERENTIAL DIAGNOSIS

When diagnosis of SAT with neck pain is considered, it should be differentiated from the other causes like acute infectious thyroiditis, hemorrhage into the cyst, painful Hashimoto's thyroiditis, thyroid malignancy (anaplastic carcinoma, lymphoma), radiation thyroiditis, and painful amiodarone-induced thyroiditis. It has also been reported following *interferon therapy* as well. Patients with SAT may present with complaints of sore throat, and many a time misdiagnosed as pharyngitis. Radioiodine scanning is an important modality in differentiating acute hemorrhage into a nodule or cyst and nonthyroidal causes. Radioiodine uptake will be normal in the unaffected area of the gland. Infectious thyroiditis is usually associated with prodromal symptoms like fever, malaise, and raised total leukocytes, and a local inflammatory response around the affected area of thyroid tissue. A nuclear uptake scan would be normal except with reduced uptake in the area of suppuration. Hashimoto's thyroiditis is rarely associated with pain, involves the whole gland with thyroglobulin, and TPO antibodies

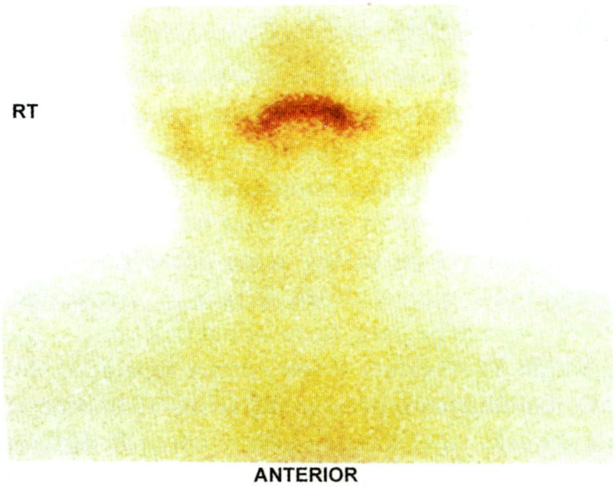

Figure 2.1: Thyroid gland barely visualized above the background and very poorly delineated salivary uptake seen

in high titers. Most important difference between the SAT and sporadic/ postpartum thyroiditis is thyroid pain; pain is almost never a feature of sporadic or postpartum thyroiditis (PPT) but commonly seen with SAT. Sporadic or PPT also has high titers of antibodies to thyroglobulin and thyroid peroxidase. ESR is markedly elevated in SAT, however, would be normal or mildly elevated in PPT.

Neck pain may initially occur on one side and later move to the opposite side (creeping thyroiditis) (Fig. 2.1).

DISCUSSION

Subacute thyroiditis is known by several names, the most common of which DeQuervain's thyroiditis. The inflammation may last for weeks to months. Subacute thyroiditis is one of the most common causes of painful thyroiditis, and accounts for about 5% of clinical thyroid disorders. Incidence of SAT reported by the Mayo clinic was 4.9 cases/100,000 from 1970 to 1997. Women are more frequently affected than men, and peak incidence is during fourth and fifth decade. It is very rare in children and in pregnancy. Granulomatous appearance of thyroid on pathologic examination is specific for SAT. Specific etiology is not clear, a viral etiology is suggested, genetic and autoimmune etiologies have also been proposed. It is more common in temperate zones in the summer months. Distinctive feature of SAT is pain in the thyroid region; pain can be severe involving the whole gland.

COURSE AND MANAGEMENT

During the acute phase, it is associated with self-limiting thyroidal pain, which usually lasts for 3–6 weeks. Thyrotoxic symptoms may be mild. Inflammatory destruction of the gland causes thyroid hormones and thyroglobulin leakage into the circulation. If the patient is symptomatic β-blockers like propranolol can be used. In SAT, antithyroid drugs have no role, as the thyroid gland is not hyperfunctioning. Pain during acute phase can be managed with nonsteroidal anti-inflammatory drugs, if pain is severe oral prednisone with up to 40 mg/day can be used, there would be dramatic relief from pain and swelling within 24–48 hours, if steroids are tapered rapidly, pain may reoccur as the inflammatory process is still active, so in general, steroids be tapered over 4–6 weeks. After several weeks in about 30–50% cases transient hypothyroidism occurs, which may last for few months, they do not need replacement if they are asymptomatic with mild TSH elevation. With overt and symptomatic hypothyroidism, treatment is justified, and might abrogate early exacerbation. Permanent hypothyroidism is relatively uncommon, but is reported to occur in 5–31% of cases. Recurrence of SAT after prolonged latency is relatively rare (4%).

KEY POINTS

We present a difficult case of recurrent thyroiditis, which did not follow the usual course, and there were multiple recurrences with intermittent normalcy. Thyroiditis often follows a predictable course, but exceptions may demand unconventional approach. Though thyroiditis rarely requires surgery this lady had to undergo surgery due to the nature of its course:

- Subacute thyroiditis is usually a self-limited inflammatory thyroid disease lasting for weeks to several months
- Thyroglobulin levels are markedly elevated
- Subacute thyroiditis usually follows a triphasic course: an initial hyperthyroid phase due to release of thyroid hormone from inflamed thyroid gland, followed by a transient hypothyroid phase and final recovery phase to euthyroid state
- Treatment with antithyroid drugs has limited role in treatment, and nonsteroidal anti-inflammatory drugs and glucocorticoids are often required to provide relief
- If symptomatic hypothyroid state ensues, replacement therapy with levothyroxine is recommended.

SUGGESTED READINGS

1. Fatourechi V, Aniszewski JP, Fatourechi GZ, et al. Clinical features and outcome of sub-acute thyroiditis in an incidence cohort: Olmsted county, Minnesota study. J Clin Endocrinol Metab. 2003;88:2100-5.
2. Lazarus J. Acute and sub-acute thyroiditis. In: Thyroid Disease Manager, Chapter 19. 2010.
3. Yamada M, Satoh T, Hashimoto K. Thyroiditis in Clinical Management of Thyroid Disease. In: Wondisford F, Radocick S (eds). Philadelphia, PA: Saunders; 2009. pp. 191-202.

CHAPTER

3

Graves' Disease

KM Prasanna Kumar

CASE PRESENTATION

A 30-year-old female married for the past 5 years, presented with the complaints of weight loss (8 kg in 3 months), hand tremor, palpitations, irritability, and heat intolerance. She also complained of increased appetite and hyperdefecation. She is a known case of bronchial asthma since childhood. She is on inhaled steroids and bronchodilators on need basis. She feels that over the past 3 months, her complexion has darkened. She and her husband are very keen to start family.

On examination, she was 156 cm tall and weighed 48 kg. Her pulse rate was 116/minute, and blood pressure 160/60 mmHg. There was no exophthalmos, and all eye movements were noted to be normal. She had diffuse enlargement of thyroid gland (two to three times the normal size) that was not tender. No bruit was overheard. No cervical lymphadenopathy or clinical signs of significant local compression were elicited. Patient's hands were moist and showed mild tremor. Examination of the heart revealed tachycardia, with no other finds of click or murmur. Examination of lungs was unremarkable. Examination of abdomen did not reveal any visceromegaly. Bowel sounds were normal. Examination of skin did not reveal any areas of hypopigmentation or loss of pigment. On onycholysis was demonstrated.

DIFFERENTIAL DIAGNOSIS

Clinical features of this patient are characteristic of thyrotoxicosis. Differential diagnosis would include:

- Graves' disease (GD)
- Acute (infectious), and subacute thyroiditis (granulomatous thyroiditis/ DeQuervain's thyroiditis)

- Toxic nodular goiter (Plummer's disease)
- Infiltrative disorders with inflammation (amyloid, sarcoid, lymphoma).

The final diagnosis of subacute granulomatous thyroiditis is based on clinical symptoms, suppressed thyrotropin (TSH), an elevated erythrocyte sedimentation rate (ESR), and/or reduced or patchy thyroid radionuclide uptake/technetium scan while hyperthyroid in the absence of thyroid antibodies. The thyroiditis may be painless as well.

INVESTIGATIONS

Clinically, this patient has features of thyrotoxicosis. The investigations should be directed to confirm the diagnosis and determine possible etiology to select appropriate mode of therapy. Preliminary investigations must include complete blood count (CBC), TSH, and iodothyronines [total and free thyroxin (T4), triiodothyronine (T3)].
Laboratory results showed:

- Serum T3: 273.8 ng/dL (normal: 70–170 ng/dL)
- Serum T4: 20 µg/dL (normal: 4.5–11.5 µg/dL)
- Serum TSH: <0.01 mIU/mL (normal: 0.3–4.0 mIU/mL)
- TSH receptor antibody (TRab): >40 IU/L (normal: <1.75 IU/L)
- ESR: 8 mm in first hour
- Tc-99 scan: Uniformly enlarged gland with increased uptake
- Thyroid ultrasonography (USG): Diffuse and uniformly enlarged with increased vascularity.

Elevated serum T3 and T4 with a low TSH is diagnostic of thyrotoxicosis. Presence TRab supports diagnosis of GD. TRab are absent in acute, and subacute thyroiditis. Imaging studies (technetium scan and thyroid USG further support diagnosis of GD.

MANAGEMENT

Patient was informed about clinical diagnosis and its verification by laboratory tests. One option is to start the patients on β-blockers, pending availability of thyroid test results. This gives patients relief from adrenergic symptoms such as palpitations, tachycardia, and tremor. However, given history of asthma in our patient, this option was considered undesirable. There are primarily three viable options that must be discussed with patient to allow them to make informed decision. These include:

- Medical management with antithyroid drugs (thionamide)

- Radioactive iodine (RAI) (I^{131})
- Surgery.

Patient preferred antithyroid drug therapy primarily driven by desire to get pregnant without too much wait. She was placed on methimazole 20 mg once daily for 6 weeks. Patient was informed about the side effects of antithyroid drug and to stop the drug in case she develops fever, sore throat, lymphadenopathy, skin rash, itching, or arthralgia/joint swellings and inform physician promptly. The white blood cell counts were performed after 3 weeks and found to be normal. After 2 months of antithyroid drug therapy, patient became euthyroid and was advised 5 mg of folic acid daily. Three months later patient conceived and was switched to propylthiouracil (PTU) 100 mg thrice a day. The serum-free T3 and T4 were monitored every 2 months and were at upper limits of normal with 300 mg/day of PTU during second and third trimesters. Patient delivered a healthy child after completing the term. The child weighed 3.2 kg and was clinically normal. The neonatal TSH was 4 mIU/mL on third day after birth. The patient continued to breastfeed the child for 1 year after delivery and she was advised to take tablet methimazole 15 mg daily and the thyroid function tests were performed periodically every 2 months and the dose of methimazole was adjusted to keep serum T3 and T4 within normal limits. After the patient stopped breastfeeding the child, she stopped the antithyroid drug therapy. Eight weeks later, she experienced the symptoms of thyrotoxicosis. The serum T3 was 224 ng/dL, serum T4 was 14.8 μg/dL, and serum TSH was <0.05 mIU/mL.

Patient was explained about the choices of therapy following relapse of Graves' thyrotoxicosis. She chose radioiodine therapy. After signed informed consent an arbitrary dose of 12 mCi of I^{131} was delivered to her. Thyroid functions were performed every 8 weeks thereafter. She was euthyroid at the end of 4 months following I^{131} therapy. She became hypothyroid at the end of 6 months with serum T4 3 μg/dL and TSH > 20 mIU/mL. She weighed 64 kg at this time. She was placed on 100 μg of levothyroxine once a day before breakfast and TSH checked after 6 weeks was 2.5 mIU/mL. The patient was advised to continue levothyroxine life long and check TSH yearly to adjust the dose of levothyroxine.

DISCUSSION

Graves' disease is an autoimmune disorder caused by stimulating antibodies against the thyrotropin receptor and is characterized by hyperthyroidism, diffuse goiter, ophthalmopathy, and rarely dermopathy. It accounts for 60–80% of all cases of hyperthyroidism, is 5–10 times more common in women than men, and is associated with a clinically evident ophthalmopathy in about 30–50% of patients. The peak incidence is observed between 40 and 60 years of age in the Western population, whereas it occurs between 30 and 50 years more frequently in our population. Thyrotoxicosis refers to clinical consequences of increased thyroid hormones in circulation, whereas hyperthyroidism refers to a state of heightened thyroid activity. The presence of ophthalmopathy or dermopathy is almost always observed in GD.

Third-generation TRab assays are available in most places. In GD, TRab should be tested before deciding whether methimazole can be stopped. TRab should be measured in pregnant women with GD to assess the risk of fetal thyrotoxicosis.

Normal ESR increased uniformly distributed tracer uptake, and increased blood flow on sonography support diagnosis of GD and effectively rule out acute of subacute thyroiditis where the tracer uptake is decrease with absent or patchy distribution. The ESR is elevated, and same is seen with high sensitivity C-reactive protein in patients with subacute thyroiditis (SAT). Positive predictive value for sonography to detect SAT is closer to 80%. The most common sonographic appearance being poor defined regions of reduced vascularity, and reduced echogenicity.

In many places I^{123} may be used to determine thyroid gland uptake, and it is no longer considered a necessary test for diagnosis particularly in areas where daily iodine intake is high and the gland likely to be loaded with stable iodine. Under these circumstances uptake may be low despite full blown hyperthyroid state. Although often stated ultrasonography reveals a uniformly enlarged thyroid gland in GD, presence of nodules need not exclude diagnosis. Occasionally hyperfunctioning nodules surrounded by hyperfunctioning paranodular tissue may be seen (Marine–Lenhart syndrome).

Management of thyrotoxicosis revolves around three main choices: antithyroid drugs (ATD), surgery and radioiodine therapy. As none of them is ideal therapy, physician should discuss all the three options with their patients and inform them about benefits and risks associated with each modality. Management should be individualized and patient's preference respected. The choice of therapy is influenced by many factors, including its cost, convenience, local cultural factors, size of the goiter, severity of disease, personal experience, as well as considerations about the risks and benefits of each form of treatment. An ideal treatment of GD would be immediate control of the disease manifestations, achieve the euthyroid state, and maintain it for life long with minimal morbidity and mortality.

Antithyroid Drugs

Antithyroid drugs inhibit the thyroid hormone synthesis by interfering with thyroid peroxidase mediated iodination of tyrosine residues in thyroglobulin. carbimazol, methimazole, and PTU are the antithyroid drugs available in India. Though the half-life of antithyroid drugs like carbimazol and methimazole are few hours, their effective life is longer and are thus given as a single daily dose, whereas PTU (half-life 1.65 hours or less) is given two to three times a day in divided dose. They are used as primary drugs in Graves' thyrotoxicosis to induce remission or prepare the patient for surgery or radioiodine therapy. Starting daily dose for Propylthiouracil could be 300 given in three divided doses compared to 15–30 mg/day of methimazole or carbimazol. In most patients euthyroid state can be reached within 4–6 weeks. If the patient fails to respond the dose may be increased. Patients on methimazole often notice bitter taste, and the drug may have to be given twice daily. It is not a bad policy to obtain CBC before therapy is started since mild leukopenia may be seen because of hyperthyroidism itself and same holds true for mild elevation in liver enzymes. One week after starting patient on ATD therapy, repeat CB and liver function tests to detect any adverse drug effects. Iodothyronines (T4 and T3) should be repeated within 2–3 weeks after initiation of therapy. If the treatment is working downward trend should be discernible at this time. There is no advantage in testing TSH at this stage since TSH suppression lasts longer. Patients may be seen at 6–8 week intervals thereafter. In about 50% of medically treated patients, a lasting remission would be expected. It is generally recommended to treat patient for 16–18 months unless contraindications prevail. The most dreaded adverse effect is agranulocytosis (0.1–0.4 %). Once agranulocytosis is detected, immediate cessation of drug therapy is warranted. For minor side effects, interclass rug substitution may be attempted under close watch. When considering stopping medical treatment, watch for normalization of T3 (T3 is first to rise and last to fall in patients with GD. Relying on T4 alone may lead to delay in diagnosis as well as premature cessation of therapy risking relapse).

In pregnant patient, specific treatment regimens have been prescribed based on the stage of pregnancy. The Endocrine Society guidelines for managing thyroid disease during pregnancy and postpartum suggests following. Antithyroid drug therapy remains the first-line choice for hyperthyroidism in pregnancy. Because PTU can rarely be associated with severe maternal liver toxicity, methimazole should be considered as an alternative after the first trimester (the two agents are equally efficacious, but first-trimester fetal exposure to methimazole has been associated with congenital abnormalities including aplasia cutis, choanal atresia). Since the ATD's cross the placenta, there is risk to fetal thyroid gland. The lowest possible dose should be used to maintain maternal free thyroxin levels at or just above the upper limit of the normal nonpregnant reference range. Serum TSH and either total or free thyroxin levels should be measured in fetal cord blood at delivery in women with active GD. The risk of fetal thyrotoxicosis from transplacental transfer of thyroid stimulating antibodies does exist in GD during pregnancy. There is also a possibility of fetal hypothyroidism from transplacental transfer of antithyroid drugs and thyroid-blocking antibodies. Maternal TRab should be measured before 22 weeks' gestation in women with GD; those with prior history of GD managed with RAI or thyroidectomy; previous neonates with GD; or previously elevated thyroid TRab. If TRab are negative in patients with prior history of treated disease, these should be repeated again between 32 and 34 week of gestation.

In pregnant women who have elevated thyroid receptor antibodies or are receiving antithyroid drugs, the possibility of risk of fetal thyroid dysfunction (as evidenced by fetal goiter, intrauterine growth restriction, hydrops, advanced bone age, tachycardia, or cardiac failure) should be assessed with ultrasound at 18–22 weeks and thereafter every 4–6 weeks or as clinically indicated. Neonatal thyrotoxicosis is generally a self-limiting disorder and clears by 11–13 weeks. If, however, signs of heart failure are noticed, treatment should be recommended and instituted.

ATD's primarily work by inhibiting thyroid hormone synthesis: They interfere with thyroid peroxidase mediated iodination of tyrosine residues in thyroglobulin. Propylthiouracil has an added advantage of reducing conversion of T4 to T3, and thus a preferred drug in T3 toxicosis. Recently, PTU has come under scrutiny because of reported hepatocellular failure associated with its use.

Surgery

Surgery for GD was largely replaced in the last few decades by radioiodine and antithyroid drugs, due to the fact that they are more safe and effective. The common indications for surgery are patient preference, presence of cold nodule, Graves' ophthalmopathy, large goiters for cosmetic reasons, allergy to antithyroid drugs, and young children below 6 years of age.

One of the meta-analysis involving 35 studies comprising 7,241 patients with a mean follow-up of 5.6 years showed persistent or recurrent hyperthyroidism occurred in 7.2% of patients. Thyroidectomy successfully treated hyperthyroidism in 92% of patients with GD and no recurrence of hyperthyroidism following total thyroidectomy. Subtotal thyroidectomy achieved a euthyroid state in almost 60% of patients of GD. Presently total thyroidectomy is preferred over subtotal thyroidectomy. Patients are advised to meet with the surgeon and discuss any risk for unwanted outcome (vocal cord injury, keloid formation, parathyroid gland injury, etc.). Once surgery has been completed, patients will require lifelong thyroid hormone replacement.

RAI Ablation

Radioactive iodine (RAI) treatment was first introduced in 1941. The use of RAI therapy as the first line of treatment has steadily increased over the years and is presently considered to be the treatment of choice in many parts of the world, for most of the patients. A recent randomized trial comparing RAI therapy with ATDs in patients with GD found that those who were smokers or had pre-existing Grave's ophthalmopathy (GO), were no more likely to experience worsening GO after RAI than after ATD therapy, but new GO occurred more frequently after RAI (38%) than with ATDs (18%). If ophthalmopathy is suspected, pretreatment with glucocorticoid must be considered.

The dosing of RAI in the therapy of Grave's thyrotoxicosis is controversial. Fixed dose of RAI appears to have good cure rate for thyrotoxicosis. Fixed dose of I^{131} ablation is a cost-effective, simple, easy, and efficient. Our own experience in the last 2 decades is that low fixed dose of I^{131} ablation in GD is as good as high dose. Our retrospective analysis compared 1 year outcomes of two fixed doses of radioiodine therapy 5 mCi (n = 77) versus 10 mCi (n = 150) in newly diagnosed women with GD who were treated from 1998 to 2006. After 1 year, the overall success rate of a single dose of radioiodine was 92.5%; 90.9% in the 5-mCi group and 93.2% in the 10-mCi group were in remission. In the 5-mCi group, 81.8% of patients were hypothyroid, 9.1% were euthyroid, and 9.1% had relapsed. The rates for the 10-mCi group were 78.6%, 14.6%, and 6.8%, respectively. This analysis showed that 10 mCi was no more effective than 5 mCi in treating female patients with GD. Kristien Boelaert studied the mortality among hyperthyroid subjects aged 40 years or older, and found that the mortality was increased during periods of thionamide treatment and after radioiodine not resulting in hypothyroidism, but not during follow-up after radioiodine-induced hypothyroidism. Studies have shown that radioiodine therapy is safe and effective even in children and adolescent.

The choice of therapy in GD varies across the globe. In response to a questionnaire in the United States, 69% of the respondents from the

American Thyroid Association suggested using RAI ablation for a patient with GD, whereas 22% of European, 22% of Chinese, 11% of Japanese, and 11% of Korean respondents selected this means of treatment.

Young females who receive RAI therapy are advised to avoid pregnancy for the following 6–12 months. Another issue that often crops up relates to compromising RAI efficacy with prior use of ATD's. This issue is far from settled.

Certainly patients must stop taking ATDs 5–7 days before anticipated RAI treatment.

CONCLUSION

Graves' disease can be easily diagnosed with disease specific laboratory and imaging work up. It is easily treated by antithyroid drugs, surgery, or RAI ablation. As none of the therapies for GD is ideal and each one has its own limitation, patient preference after discussion is the best approach. Antithyroid drugs for 12–18 months can induce remission in nearly half the patients. Antithyroid drugs remain the cornerstone of therapy in GD during pregnancy. Surgery is a safe alternative in experienced hands, and results are evident in very short period. Since most patients get total thyroidectomy, lifelong replacement with thyroid hormone becomes mandatory. Radioactive iodine therapy is one of the common therapies for Graves' thyrotoxicosis and is the preferred first line of therapy. Radioactive iodine is a safe, simple and economical therapy for GD. Hypothyroidism is a limiting factor in RAI for GD. Except pregnant and lactating women, and those desiring pregnancy within 6 months and children <6 years of age, there is no absolute contraindication to RAI.

KEY POINTS

- Graves' disease is a common endocrine disorder among young females
- Graves' disease has specific hormonal, immunological, and imaging profile that makes it easy to differentiate from thyroiditis
- Several treatment options exist, and treatment plan should be discussed with each patient
- Graves' disease during pregnancy is not treated with RAI. Medical therapy is the mainstay. Surgical option can be considered in late second and third trimesters
- Treatment preferences vary across globe.

SUGESSTED READINGS

1. Barbesino G, Tomer Y. Clinical utility of TSH receptor antibodies. J Clin Endocrinol Metab. 2013;98: 2247-55.
2. Boelaert K, Maisonneuve P, Torlinska B, et al. Comparison of mortality in hyperthyroidism during periods of treatment with thionamide and after radioiodine. J Clin Endocrinol Metab. 2013;98:1869-82.
3. Brent GA. Clinical practice, Graves' disease. N Engl J Med. 2008;358:2594-605.
4. De Groot L, Abalovich M, Alexander EK, et al. Practice guidelines management of thyroid dysfunction during pregnancy and postpartum: an Endocrine Society clinical practice guideline. J Clin Endocrinol Metab. 2012;97:2543-65.
5. Hyperthyroidism. Cooper DS. Lancet. 2003;362(9382):459-68.
6. Kumar P, Prasad S. Comparison of efficacy of two fixed doses of I^{131} radioiodine therapy (5 vs. 10 mCi) in female patients with Graves' disease. Abstract # 40. The 82nd Annual Meeting of the American Thyroid Association (ATA) Annual Meeting, Québec City, Québec, from September 19–23, 2012.

CHAPTER

4

Vanishing Pituitary Tumor

Vinay Dipali, Vageesh Ayyar S

CASE PRESENTATION

A 32-year-old male was referred to endocrine service for evaluation and further management of pituitary mass. He presented with acute history of headache, recurrent vomiting, easy fatigability, and diffuse aches, and pains. He also complained of nausea, reduced appetite, and loss of libido, polyuria, and polydipsia. He had no comorbidities and no significant past history except for one episode of febrile illness 2 weeks prior to the presentation that subsided spontaneously. No history of hospitalization in the past. General physical and systemic examination was normal with no localizing signs.

DIFFERENTIAL DIAGNOSIS

In a patient with known lesion in sellar/suprasellar region and constellation of symptoms described above, following considerations are important to plan diagnostic approach as well as immediate management:

- Pituitary adenoma/infiltrative disorder/inflammatory lesion/infectious process
- Pituitary apoplexy
- Hypopituitarism
    - Hypogonadism
    - Hypoadrenalism
- Diabetes insipidus.

INVESTIGATIONS

- Fasting blood glucose: 84 mg/dL (normal: 75–100 mg/dL)
- Hemoglobin: 14.1 g%
- White blood cell count: 8,110 (normal differential count)
- Differential count: Normal
- Erythrocyte sedimentation rate: 16 mm in first hour
- Serum creatinine: 0.7 mg/dL
- Serum sodium: 142 mmol/L
- Serum potassium: 4.2 mmol/L
- Liver function studies: Normal
- Routine urinalysis: Normal
- Workup for fever: Normal
- 24-hour fluid intake/output: 6 L/5.5 L
- Morning (8 AM) plasma cortisol: 0.8 ng/dL (normal: 7–20 μg/dL)
- Thyroid-stimulating hormone (TSH): 0.09 μU/mL (normal: 0.2–4.5 μU/mL)
- Free thyroxine (FT4): 0.6 ng/dL (normal: 0.8–2.1 ng/dL)
- Total plasma testosterone: <1 ng/mL (normal: 350–1,050 ng/dL)
- Follicle stimulating hormone: 0.9 mIU/mL
- Luteinizing hormone: <0.1 IU/mL
- Prolactin: 28.2 ng/mL (normal: 3–18 ng/mL)
- Imaging studies
    - Magnetic resonance imaging (MRI) of pituitary: Well-defined homogenously enhancing lesion, not separately visualized from the pituitary gland, causing expansion of sella with suprasellar extension and abutting the optic chiasm (Fig. 4.1).

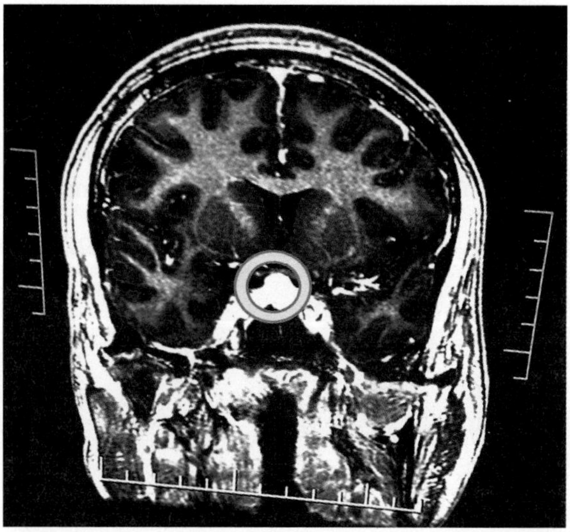

Figure 4.1: Post contrast MRI at diagnosis. Note the thickened stalk and homogenously enhancing pituitary

DIAGNOSIS

Combined pituitary hormone deficiency with diabetes insipidus: lymphocytic hypophysitis.

MANAGEMENT

Based on the clinical, biochemical, and MRI findings, a diagnosis of lymphocytic hypophysitis was made. Patient was started on replacement doses of thyroxine (1.6 μg/kg/day), hydrocortisone (12 mg/m^2/day) and testosterone (250 mg every 3 weeks, IM). Patient was asked to follow-up every month with hormonal assessment. We could see the recovery of pituitary function on follow-up, testosterone and thyroxine replacement were stopped and hydrocortisone dose was tapered and stopped. Patient is currently off all medications with a totally normal pituitary profile. He required replacement for a total duration of 6 months (including the time required for tapering). His repeat MRI showed a normal pituitary with no changes in signal intensities (Fig. 4.2). Patient will be asked to follow-up with periodic pituitary function assessment.

DISCUSSION

Inflammatory involvement of pituitary gland (hypophysitis) is relatively uncommon and mimics pituitary adenoma clinically and radiologically. Treatment options for these two diagnoses vary and the two can be differentiated unequivocally only by tissue biopsy. Lymphocytic hypophysitis

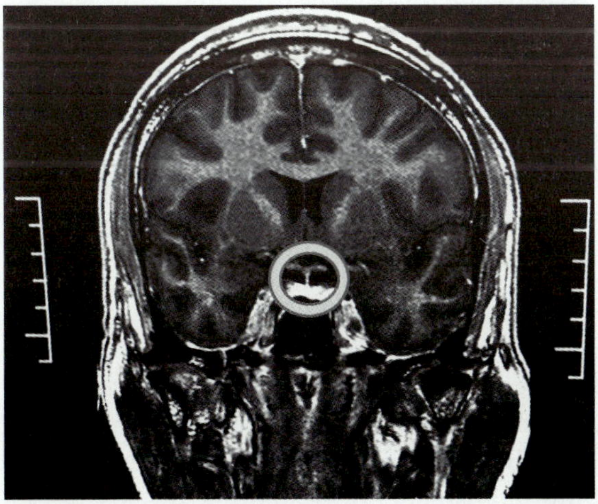

Figure 4.2: MRI at follow up visit. Note the resolution of mass and clear visualisation of the stalk

is an inflammatory disorder and presumed to have autoimmune basis. Autoimmune hypophysitis was first described in 1962 by Goudie and Pinkerton. They reported a 22-year-old woman, 14 months after her second child birth. She died 8 hours following appendectomy, presumably compounded by adrenal insufficiency. Her pituitary gland showed lymphocytic infiltration.

Definition

Currently three forms of hypophysitis are recognized: lymphocytic hypophysitis, granulomatous hypophysitis, and xanthomatous hypophysitis. Each of these may develop de novo or secondary to a systemic process. Lymphocytic hypophysitis being relatively common has received the most attention. Idiopathic granulomatous hypophysitis was first described in 1908, while Xanthomatous hypophysitis was described first in 1998.

Lymphocytic hypophysitis is further subdivided based on affected anatomical target:

1. Lymphocytic adenohypophysitis (LAH) when only anterior pituitary is involved.
2. Lymphocytic infundibuloneurohypophysitis (LINH) when there is exclusive involvement of pituitary stalk and posterior pituitary.
3. Lymphocytic infundibulopanhypophysitis (LIPH) that has features of both anterior and posterior pituitary involvement.

Epidemiology

Lymphocytic hypophysitis is a relatively rare disease with a reported incidence of 1 in 9 million individuals (<1% of unselected samples obtained at surgery). Majority of cases reported are females though significant proportion of men have been reported as well (23%). It is seen most often in the later stages of pregnancy or immediate postpartum period, and less often in the peripubertal and postmenopausal period. Mean age at diagnosis is around 35 years in females and 45 years in males. As opposed to lymphocytic hypophysitis, there is no predominant female predilection in granulomatous and xanthomatous types.

Pathology

In lymphocytic hypophysitis, pituitary histopathology reveals diffuse inflammation with widespread infiltration by inflammatory cells comprising polymorphs, lymphocytes, plasma cells, histiocytes, and occasional eosinophils. Immunohistochemical staining reveals presence of both B (CD20 positive) and T (CD3 positive) cells admixed with macrophages

(CD 68 positive). In granulomatous hypophysitis, histiocytes and multinucleated giant cells and granulomas would be seen. In xanthomatous hypophysitis, cystic areas interspersed with foamy histiocytes are seen.

Although considered an autoimmune process (association with other autoimmune diseases, inflammatory/immune cell infiltration on histopathology), no specific antigen or antigens have been identified. Antibodies against pituitary and hypothalamic tissue, hormones secreted by the pituitary, transcription factors involved in pituitary development, and nonpituitary tissues (thyroid, testis) have been reported. Similar antibodies have been reported in certain individuals without evidence of hypophysitis. Thus, it is not recommended to include these antibodies in the formal evaluation of patients.

Progress in understanding of pathogenesis of hypophysitis was limited due to nonavailability of animal model. The development of mouse model should lead to better understanding. However, it is not always easy to translate mice studies to human biology. Recently increasing number of hypophysitis and hypothalamitis are being reported following introduction of cytotoxic T-lymphocyte antigen-4 (CTLA-4) blockers (ipilimumab) to treat malignant melanoma.

Clinical Features

Symptoms/presentation in those with lymphocytic hypophysitis may be related in majority of the cases to mass effect from expanding pituitary gland and stalk (58%). Symptoms include headache, visual field defects and decreased visual acuity. Second common presentation relates to consequences arising from deficiency of anterior pituitary hormones (44%); ACTH deficiency being most predominant (32% of cases), followed by TSH deficiency (15%), and gonadotropin deficiency (14%). There are no precise data available on growth hormone deficiency. Third presentation relates to diabetes insipidus (31%) consequent to stalk involvement disrupting axonal transport of antidiuretic hormone from the hypothalamic nuclei to the posterior pituitary. Some patients present with symptoms of hyperprolactinemia (17–23%).

ACTH deficiency is earliest functional alteration reported in patients with lymphocytic hypophysitis.

Diagnosis

Diagnosis requires high index of suspicion and thorough evaluation of clinical setting and risk factors. Evaluation requires full assessment of both anterior and posterior pituitary functions. Once biochemical evaluation is complete, imaging of sellar and suprasellar structures is necessary. Whereas diabetes insipidus is very common in LIPH and LINH, it is less frequent with LAH. Females predominate in LAH while LIPH and LINH are seen more in men. Ultimately the distinctions rests on histopathology of tissue obtained at biopsy or surgery.

Immunophenotyping is not recommended since markers cited in literature are very nonspecific, and also do not segregate according to the region of pituitary affected.

Imaging

Findings on MRI in patients with lymphocytic hypophysitis may overlap with those seen in patients with pituitary adenoma. Enlargement of the pituitary gland with thickening of infundibulum extending into suprasellar area is seen in almost 80% of cases. After contrast administration there is marked early and homogenous enhancement often involving the dura (*dural tail*). A strong and homogenous enhancement of the anterior pituitary, similar to the cavernous sinus, is more suggestive of an inflammatory infiltrative process such as lymphocytic hypophysitis rather than a macroadenoma. Macroadenomas enhance less or more slowly than the normal pituitary on dynamic MRI. Certain radiological features may help differentiate hypophysitis from an adenoma (Table 4.1). It should be noted that there may be lack of radiological abnormalities in a very small percentage of patients, and also abnormalities may evolve slowly after hormonal abnormalities have appeared.

Even when using modern MRI studies, approximately 40% of the cases are misdiagnosed preoperatively as pituitary adenomas. Hence, the gold standard for diagnosis of lymphocytic hypophysitis is the pituitary biopsy.

Lymphocytic hypophysitis may coexist with other pituitary lesions such as germinoma, pituitary apoplexy, and pituitary adenoma. These lesions may be encountered in associated systemic pathology such as Wegener's granulo-

TABLE 4.1: Magnetic resonance imaging features: lymphocytic hypophysitis versus pituitary adenoma

Feature	Lymphocytic hypophysitis	Pituitary adenoma
Asymmetric mass	No	Yes
Intact sellar floor	Yes	±
Suprasellar extension	Yes	±
Stalk thickening	Yes	No
Stalk displacement	No	±
Homogeneous enhancement	Yes	No
Loss of posterior pituitary bright spot	Yes	No

matosis, Langerhans histiocytosis, lymphocytic thyroiditis, sarcoidosis, tuberculosis, and other bacterial, viral or fungal processes.

MANAGEMENT

Although the transition is often from symptoms of mass effect to development of hypopituitarism, some cases may show spontaneous, partial, or full recovery. About 10% cases eventually develop the "empty sella syndrome." Death is rare, but reported in some cases and is possibly related to unattended glucocorticoid deficiency.

During the phase of hypopituitarism, patients will require hormone replacement hydrocortisone, thyroxine, and testosterone. In those with diabetes insipidus, 1-desamino-8-d-arginine vasopressin must be provided to avoid serious water and electrolyte disturbances. Up to 70% of cases require life-long hormone replacement. Periodic monitoring is necessary. Use of steroids remains controversial since resolution has not been uniformly reported, even when using high doses. Furthermore perils of chronic glucocorticoid replacement must be weighed when contemplating large dose steroids.

This case is remarkable for efficacy of glucocorticoids in mitigating hormone.

Deficits as well as resolution of sellar and supra sellar abnormalities noted on the MRI. It serves as a reminder that clinical judgment sometimes trumps trends in literature.

Surgery may be needed when the mass is rapidly increasing and leading to neurovascular compromise. Radiotherapy has been used in a small number of cases.

KEY POINTS

- Lymphocytic hypophysitis is rare but increasingly recognized clinical entity
- It should be considered in the differential diagnosis of any nonsecretory pituitary mass, especially if presenting during pregnancy or postpartum
- Tissue histopathology (obtained at biopsy or surgery) remains the most definitive way of establishing the diagnosis
- Treatment is dictated by the clinical presentation
- Immunophenotyping is not helpful in diagnosis at the present state of art
- When hypopituitarism is suspected, it must be treated actively, and patient monitored periodically for any recovery. Amongst the hormone replacements, sex steroids are least necessary particularly when considering that acute sickness is often associated with reversible secondary hypogonadism.

SUGGESTED READINGS

1. Falorni A, Minarelli V1, Bartoloni E, et al. Diagnosis and classification of autoimmune hypophysitis. Autoimmune Rev. 2014;13(4-5):412-6.
2. Hindocha A, Chudhary BR, Kearney T, et al. Lymphocytic Hypophysitis in males. Case Reports. J Clin Neurosci. 2013;20:743-5.
3. Howlett TA, Levy MJ, Robertson IJ, et al. How reliably can autoimmune hypophysitis be diagnosed without pituitary biopsy. Clin Endocrinol (Oxf). 2010;73:18-21.
4. Khare S, Jagtap VS, Budyal SR, et al. Primary (autoimmune) hypophysitis: a single centre experience. Printed online: Pituitary, December 28, 2013.
5. Ole-Petter R, Hamnvik, Anna R Laury, et al. Lymphocytic hypophysitis with diabetes insipidus in a young man. Nat Rev Endocrinol. 2010;6:464-70.
6. Torino F, Barnabei A, De Vecchis L, et al. Hypophysitis induced by monoclonal antibodies to cytotoxic T lymphocyte antigen 4: challenges from a new cause of rare disease. Oncologist. 2012;17:525-35.

CHAPTER

5

Unusual Cause of Hypocalcemia in a Young Male

Vijaykumar S Bhavi, Belinda George, Ganapathi Bantwal

CASE PRESENTATION

A 20-year-old male who was diagnosed to have seizure disorder for past 2 years presented with refractory seizures associated with abnormal posturing of both upper limbs and lower limbs. His current treatment included 200 mg of phenytoin/day. He also complained of hard bony lesions present over the right elbow from childhood and his scholastic performance was below average.

On clinical examination he was found to have short stature with a height standard deviation score (SDS) of 3.8 and features suggestive of Albright's hereditary osteodystrophy (AHO) phenotype–short stubby fingers, potter's thumb, short 4th metacarpal (Archibald's sign), and short 4th metatarsal. Both Chvostek's and Trousseau's signs were positive. He was also found to have gum hypertrophy, widely spaced teeth and subcutaneous calcifications over the right elbow. The rest of the systemic examination was normal (Figs 5.1 and 5.2).

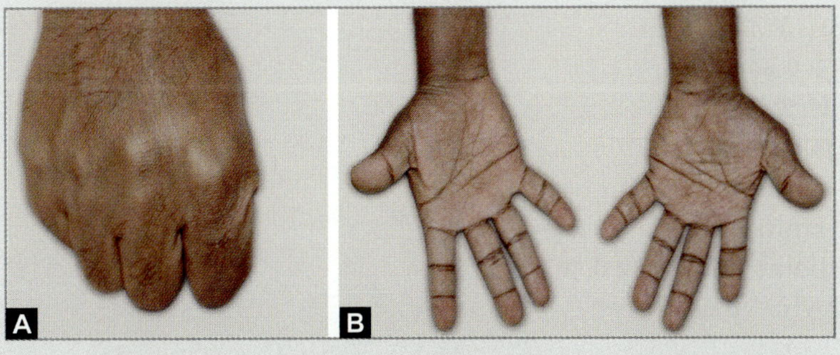

Figure 5.1: Albright's hereditary osteodystrophy phenotype. **(A)** Archibald's sign—dimple over the fourth knuckle. **(B)** Short stubby fingers and potter's thumb

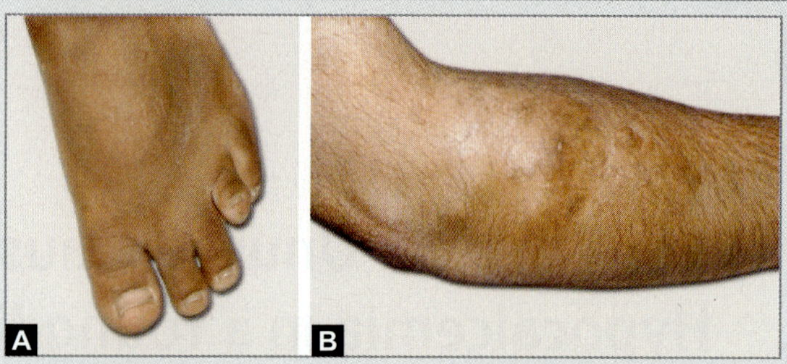

Figure 5.2: Albright's hereditary osteodystrophy phenotype. **(A)** Short 4th and 5th toe. **(B)** Subcutaneous calcifications over the right elbow joint

PROBABLE DIAGNOSIS

1. Pseudohypoparathyroidism (PHP)
2. Phenytoin induced vitamin D deficiency—rickets.

INVESTIGATIONS

- Serum calcium: 4.6 mg/dL
- Serum phosphorus: 7.2 mg/dL
- Serum albumin: 3.4 g/dL
- Serum alkaline phosphatase: 197 U/L
- PTH: 214 pg/mL
- 25-hydroxy vitamin D: 12.95 ng/dL
- ABG: Normal
- FBS: 69 mg/dL
- TSH: 31.5 mU/mL
- FT4: 0.64 ng/dL
- FSH: 2.98 mIU/L
- LH: 3.23 mIU/L
- Testosterone: 4.39 ng/mL
- 24 hours urine Ca: 39 mg
- 24 hours urine PO_4: 0.46 mg
- HbA1c: 5.0%.

RADIOLOGICAL INVESTIGATIONS

See Figs 5.3 and 5.4.

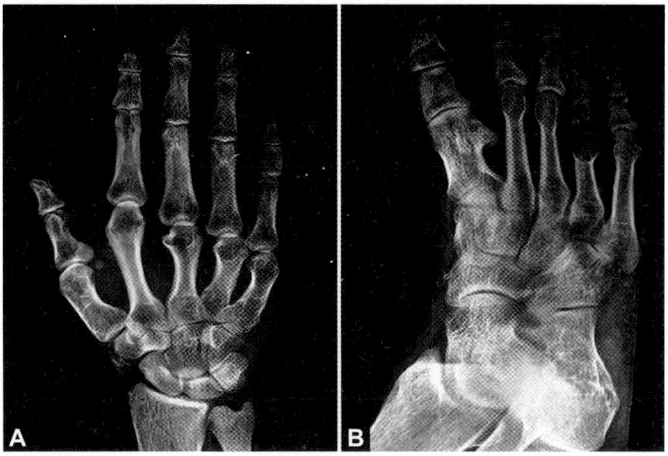

Figure 5.3: X-rays. **(A)** Short 4th metacarpal. **(B)** Short 4th metatarsal

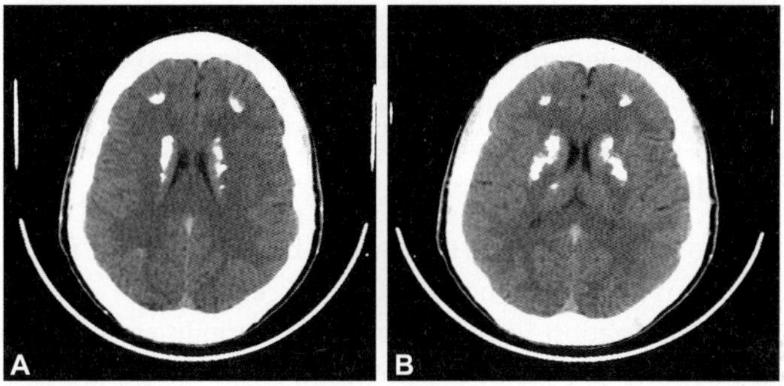

Figure 5.4: CT brain plain: extensive cerebral and basal ganglia calcification with diffuse calvarial thickening

MANAGEMENT

Biochemical evaluation confirmed hypocalcemia and hyperphosphatemia suggestive of hypoparathyroidism. Patient also had normal renal functions with elevated levels of parathyroid hormone (PTH). This biochemical finding along with presence of AHO phenotype confirms the diagnosis of PHP. Patient also had hypothyroidism with elevated TSH levels and low free T4 levels. There were no other endocrine defects (gonadotropin, testosterone and prolactin were all within the normal reference range).

Patient initially received calcium gluconate infusion for symptomatic hypocalcemia during hospital stay followed by oral calcium carbonate (2 g/day) in four divided doses along with oral calcitriol (1 μg/day). The antiepileptic drug was changed to levetiracetam in view of known side effects of phenytoin on bone and mineral metabolism. Patient was also started on thyroxine replacement for hypothyroidism.

On follow-up, the dose of calcium and calcitriol were adjusted to maintain calcium levels around 8–8.5 mg/dL. Urinary calcium excretion was also monitored to ensure hypercalciuria is absent. Currently the patient has achieved a satisfactory calcium-phosphate homeostasis with 0.5 µg/day of calcitriol, 1.5 g of calcium carbonate, and 100 µg of levothyroxine.

DISCUSSION

Pseudohypoparathyroidism is a rare genetic disorder characterized by hypocalcemia and hyperphosphatemia in presence of elevated PTH levels that occurs due to resistance to the action of PTH. This condition was originally described by Fuller Albright in 1942 among a group of patients with certain phenotypic features like short stature, brachydactyly, mental retardation, and obesity along with hypocalcemia and hyperphosphatemia. This clinical picture is currently described as the AHO phenotype and includes short stature, obesity, round facies, mental retardation, ectopic calcification, and brachydactyly. These patients were also demonstrated to have resistance to other hormones like thyrotropin and gonadotropins.

Pathophysiology

The resistance to PTH action in PHP seems to be limited to the proximal renal tubule. The actions of PTH on bone and distal renal tubule are normal. This results in the combination of biochemical abnormalities seen in PHP. The predominant actions of PTH at the proximal renal tubule are activation of 1α-hydroxylase and phosphate excretion. The predominant actions of PTH at the distal tubule and skeleton are calcium reabsorption and resorption of bones, respectively. Hyperphosphatemia occurs predominantly because of the compromised phosphaturic action of PTH at the proximal renal tubule and partly due to the normal resorptive action of PTH on the skeleton. The levels of 1,25 $(OH)_2$ vitamin D are reduced due to lack of PTH-mediated activation of 1α-hydroxylase enzyme. The reduced levels of 1,25 $(OH)_2$ vitamin D levels leads to reduced intestinal calcium absorption and contributes to the hypocalcemia. The resorptive actions of PTH on bone and the normal PTH-mediated reabsorption of calcium at the distal tubule may lessen the severity of hypocalcemia and is considered to be the reason for absence of symptomatic hypocalcemia in some of these patients, and this also explains the absence of hypercalciuria and low incidence of renal failure and kidney stones seen in PHP.

Patients may present with classical signs of hypocalcemia like muscle spasms and tetany, or rarely with seizures or movement disorders secondary to both hypocalcemia and the associated intracerebral calcification. The electroencephalogram may show epileptiform activity which responds to antiepileptic therapy, and this may lead to a delay in the accurate diagnosis. The defect causing PHP has been localized to a heterozygous inactivating mutation in the gene encoding for the G-stimulatory protein alpha subunit (GNAS). The mechanism of G-stimulatory protein alpha subunit (Gsα) mediated hormonal action is described in figure 5.5. Inactive Gsα is normally present in the cell as a basal assembled complex with βγ subunits. Once PTH binds to its receptor, PTHR1, the GDP molecule attached to the α-subunit is replaced with a GTP molecule. This leads to dissociation of the α-subunit from the basal assembled complex and induces downstream effects, the predominant one being cAMP generation. This action is terminated by the intrinsic GTP hydrolase activity that allows the complex to return to its original assembled state. A defective Gsα leads to the resistance seen in PHP patients, not just to PTH, but also to other hormones like TSH and gonadotropins.

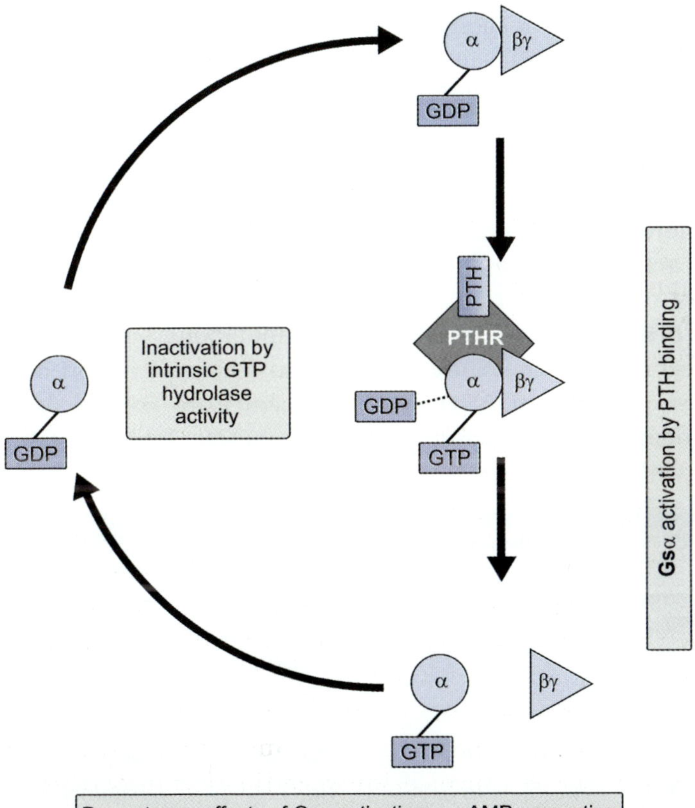

GTP, guanosine triphosphate; GDP, guanosine diphosphate; PTH, parathyroid hormone; PTHR, parathyroid hormone receptor; TSH, thyroid stimulating hormone.

Figure 5.5: Parathyroid hormone mediated Gsα action

Classification

Based on the renal response to exogenously administered PTH (Ellsworth-Howard test), PHP is classified into two main types. The Ellsworth-Howard test is carried out by measuring urinary phosphate and urinary cAMP levels following administration of PTH. In PHP type 1 (PHP 1), both urinary cAMP and phosphate responses are blunted, but in PHP type 2 (PHP 2), only urinary phosphate excretion is blunted and the cAMP response is normal. Pseudohypoparathyroidism type 1 is further categorized based on the clinical phenotype and genetic defects involved.

Pseudohypoparathyroidism types 1a and 1c are identical in their clinical and biochemical characteristics, such that both syndromes exhibit the classic AHO phenotype and also have PTH resistance characterized by hypocalcemia and hyperphosphatemia. In PHP 1a, the Gsα activity is reduced in erythrocytes; however, this reduction in Gsα activity is absent in PHP 1c. The presence of normal Gsα activity in erythrocytes (assay using nonhydrolysable GTP analogs rather than agonist-induced receptor activation) suggests that the mutations responsible in PHP 1c interferes with α-subunit coupling with G-protein-coupled receptors. Pseudohypoparathyroidism type 1b is characterized by occurrence of PTH resistance; however, they lack the AHO phenotype that is classically associated with the disease. Pseudo-pseudohypoparathyroidism (PPHP) is another variant where the typical AHO phenotype and skeletal deformities may be present, but they lack any biochemical abnormality as there is no resistance to PTH or other hormones. Progressive osseous heteroplasia (POH) may be considered as a distant variant of PHP as it shares identical genetic mutations, but has neither the biochemical nor clinical features that are classical for PHP. It is thought to be more severe form of AHO with significant extra skeletal ossification involving deep connective tissue and skeletal muscle. Table 5.1 summarizes the classification of PHP type 1.

TABLE 5.1: Variants of pseudohypoparathyroidism

	AHO phenotype	PTH resistance	Other hormonal resistance	GNAS allele origin
PHP 1a	Yes	Yes	TSH, Gn, GHRH, glucagon	Maternal
PHP 1b	No	Yes	TSH	Imprinting defect—maternal
PHP 1c	Yes	Yes	TSH, Gn	Maternally
PPHP	Yes	No	No	Paternal
POH	No	No	No	Paternal

AHO, Albright's hereditary osteodystrophy; GNAS, guanine nucleotide binding protein, alpha stimulating; PHP, pseudohypoparathyroidism; PPHP, pseudo-pseudohypoparathyroidism; POH, progressive osseous heteroplasia; PTH, parathyroid hormone; GHRH, growth-hormone-releasing hormone; TSH, thyroid-stimulating hormone.

Genetics

The genetic defect associated with PHP has been localized to the GNAS complex located in chromosome 20q, which is the region that codes for Gsα. The Gsα coding region of GNAS is biallelically expressed in most tissues in the body except renal proximal tubule, thyroid, pituitary, and gonads. The haploinsufficiency of Gsα is considered to be responsible for the AHO phenotype, and is seen in PHP 1a, PHP 1c, and PPHP. In all these conditions, a GNAS coding region mutation has been demonstrated leading to AHO phenotype. The resistance to hormones occurs only if the mutation is maternally inherited, as paternal Gsα is normally silenced in these tissues (proximal kidney tubule, thyroid, pituitary, and gonads). Therefore, paternal inheritance of this mutation will lead to PPHP, i.e. presence of AHO phenotype without the typical hormonal resistance.

Diagnosis

The diagnosis of PHP is largely clinical, and in patients with hypocalcemia and hyperphosphatemia along with normal renal functions, an elevated PTH is suggestive of PHP. The presence of AHO phenotype confirms the diagnosis. The Ellsworth-Howard test, which measures urinary cAMP and phosphate response to IV PTH infusion, may be used for additional confirmation. Molecular studies may be carried out for identifying the mutation in GNAS if facilities are available. All patients with PHP 1a should be actively screened for other endocrinopathies.

Treatment and follow-up

Treatment of PHP is similar to other forms of hypoparathyrodism and includes active vitamin D (calcitriol) and oral calcium supplements. The dose adjustment should be done not just to maintain normocalcemia but also to normalize the PTH levels. This is important to avoid the long-term exposure of bones to elevated PTH levels that may induce "hyperparathyroid bone disease." As the action of PTH at the distal tubule is preserved, the risk of hypercalciuria and nephrocalcinosis is less in PHP patients, allowing aggressive replacement of active vitamin D and calcium. Hypothyroidism and hypogonadism should be identified and treated as indicated. The short stature seen in PHP is multifactorial. The haploinsufficiency of Gsα (premature apoptosis of growth plate chondrocytes), hypogonadism (lack of pubertal growth spurt), vitamin D and calcium deficiency, and GH deficiency (resistance to GHRH) are all likely to contribute to the short stature. There is not enough evidence to support GH therapy in short stature associated with

PHP, and even in those patients with documented GH deficiency (GHD), the relative contribution of GHD to short stature is uncertain.

Patients should be monitored annually with biochemical tests which include calcium, albumin, phosphate, PTH, 24-hour urinary calcium excretion and TSH. In children with PHP, monitoring growth velocity and pubertal development and progression is essential. As they are prone to obesity, weight and body mass index should be checked at every visit and appropriate life style modification introduced when necessary.

KEY POINTS

- Pseudohypoparathyroidism (PHP) includes a rare heterogeneous group of disorders characterized by hypocalcemia, hyperphosphatemia, and elevated parathyroid hormone (PTH) levels with or without the classical AHO phenotype
- The categorization of PHP is based on whether the underlying mutation is a GNAS structural or expression defect, the difference in tissue expression (biallelic or imprinted) and parental transmission of the mutation
- Patients with PHP-I should be routinely screened and treated for any additional endocrinopathy, particularly hypothyroidism and hypogonadism
- Treatment with active vitamin D and oral calcium supplementation should be given and the dose should be adjusted to maintain calcium and PTH levels in the normal range
- Patients with PHP should be monitored annually for blood biochemistries (PTH, calcium, phosphate, TSH), 24-hour urinary calcium excretion, and special attention must be given in children to height, growth velocity, and pubertal development.

SUGGESTED READINGS

1. Chase LR, Melson GL, Aurbach GD. Pseudohypoparathyroidism: defective excretion of 3¢, 5¢-AMP in response to parathyroid hormone. J Clin Invest. 1969;48:1832-44.
2. Kelsey G. Imprinting on chromosome 20: tissue-specific imprinting and imprinting mutations in the GNAS locus. Am J Med Genet C Semin Med Genet. 2010;154C(3):377-86.
3. Kronenberg. Williams Textbook of Endocrinology, 12th edition.
4. Mann JB, Alterman S, Hills AG. Albright's hereditary osteodystrophy comprising pseudohypoparathyroidism and pseudo-pseudohypoparathyroidism. With a report of two cases representing the complete syndrome occurring in successive generations. Ann Intern Med. 1962;56:315-42.
5. Mantovani G. Pseudohypoparathyroidism: Diagnosis and Treatment. J Clin Endocrinol Metab. 2011; 96:3020-30.

CHAPTER

6

Non-parathyroid-mediated Hypercalcemia

Rajesh Rajput, Vasudha Goel

CASE PRESENTATION

A 68-year-old male, chronic smoker for 40 years, and a known case of chronic obstructive pulmonary disease, presented to emergency department with chief complaint of recurrent episodes of confusion. On further questioning he reported persistent cough with scanty sputum, generalized weakness, fatigue and loss of appetite gradually worsening over the past 6 months. He further reported unintentional weight loss of around 10 kg during past 2 months, constipation, increased thirst, and excessive urination. He denied any significant medical history in past.

On examination the patient appeared dehydrated and cachectic. He was conscious but confused. His blood pressure was normal (130/85 mmHg.) and heart rate was 96 beats/minute. He was pale and fingers revealed clubbing that had progressed rapidly. His HEENT (head, eyes, ear, nose, and throat) examination was remarkable for palpable lymph nodes bilaterally in supraclavicular region. Neurological examination did not reveal any focal motor or sensory localizing findings. Cardiac examination was unremarkable except for grade II/VI ejection systolic murmur at the base of heart. Peripheral vascular examination did not reveal any pathological findings.

Respiratory/pulmonary examination revealed dullness to percussion and decreased breath sounds on auscultation in left lower thoracic region. Examination of abdomen did not reveal any visceromegaly.

LABORATORY INVESTIGATIONS

- Hemoglobin: 9 g/dL (normal: 13–15 g/dL)
- White blood cell: 9,200/mm^3 (normal: 4,000–7,000 mm^3) (neutrophils 76%)
- Blood urea nitrogen (BUN): 44 mg/dL (normal: 10–20 mg/dL)

- Creatinine: 1.4 mg/dL (normal: 0.7–1.0 mg/dL)
- Sodium: 148 mEq/L (normal: 138–145 mEq/L)
- Potassium: 4.4 mEq/L (normal: 3.5–5.0 mEq/L)
- Chloride: 102 mEq/L (normal: 95–102 mEq/L)
- Calcium: 12.8 mg/dL (normal: 8.5–10.2 mg/dL)
- Phosphorus: 2.6 mg/dL (normal: 3.0–4.5 mg/dL)
- Total proteins: 6.6 g/dL (normal: 4.5–6.5 g/dL)
- Albumin: 3.1 g/dL (normal: 3.5–4.5 g/dL)
- Aspartate aminotransferase: 41 U/L
- Alanine aminotransferase: 37 U/L
- Alkaline phosphatase: 124 IU/L
- Glucose: 156 mg/dL
- Erythrocyte sedimentation rate: 30 mm in first hour
- Urinalysis: Unremarkable. No Bence Jones Proteins
- Electrocardiogram: Prolonged QT interval
- Chest X-ray: Homogeneous opacity in left lower lung field
- Chest CT: Homogeneous mass 3 cm in diameter in left lower lobe
- Atelectasis of left lower lobe along with a 2-cm mediastinal lymph node
- Fine needle aspiration cytology (lung mass): Squamous cell carcinoma.

Special Studies

1. Intact parathyroid hormone (PTH): 24 pg/mL (normal: 15–50 pg/mL)
2. PTH-rp: 132.2 pmol/L (normal: 13.8–55.3 pmol/L).

Patient was initially managed with intravenous fluids and diuretic followed by a zoledronic acid infusion. Patient regained complete consciousness and orientation and received on chemoradiotherapy. During next 3 months, he had recurrent episodes of confusion and disorientation that were managed similarly. He expired 6 months later. No autopsy was obtained.

DIFFERENTIAL DIAGNOSIS

Here we present a case of carcinoma of lung with hypercalcemia. For diagnostic purposes, it is useful to differentiate two categories of hypercalcemia. Those resulting primarily from hypersecretion of parathyroid hormone (PTH-mediated) and those where hypercalcemia occurs despite appropriate suppression of PTH secretion (non-PTH mediated).

It should be noted that primary hyperparathyroidism might coexist independently in many cases with malignancies. Whether this represents any causal relationship remains unclear.

TABLE 6.1: Causes of non-PTH-mediated hypercalcemia

1. Malignancy
   - Humoral hypercalcemia of malignancy (PTH-rp mediated)-solid tumors like lung, head and neck squamous cell carcinomas, renal cell carcinomas
   - Local osteolysis (cytokine mediated): Multiple myeloma, breast cancer
2. Vitamin D mediated
   - Vitamin D intoxication
   - Granulomatous diseases like tuberculosis, berylliosis, sarcoidosis
   - Hodgkin's lymphoma
3. Medications
   - Thiazide diuretics (mild)
   - Milk-Alkali syndrome (from calcium carbonate containing antacids)
   - Vitamin A intoxication (including isotretinoin analogs)
4. Other endocrine diseases
   - Thyrotoxicosis
   - Adrenal insufficiency
   - Pheochromocytoma
5. Genetic
   - William's syndrome
   - Jansen's metaphyseal chondrodysplasia
6. Others
   - Immobilization with high bone turnover as in Paget's disease, children

The case presented here is an example on non-PTH mediated hypercalcemia as reflected by low normal iPTH.

Causes of non-PTH mediated hypercalcemia are summarized in table 6.1.

APPROACH TO HYPERCALCEMIA

Evaluation of a patient with hypercalcemia includes a careful history and physical examination focusing on clinical manifestations of hypercalcemia such as fatigue, muscle weakness, confusion or coma; back pain, bone pain or fractures; kidney stones, polyuria, polydipsia; nausea, anorexia, weight loss, constipation, abdominal pain. Risk factors for malignancy should be assessed and patients should be enquired about any cough, dyspnea, ulcer disease, tumors of head and neck, any recent mammograms or chest radiographs. Other important elements in the medical history include inquiry regarding ingestion of medications, like vitamin A or D, calcium preparations, lithium, thiazides, and family history of hypercalcemia associated conditions or other endocrinopathies.

Concentrations of total serum calcium in normal serum generally range between 8.5 and 10.5 mg/dL and levels above this are considered to be consistent with hypercalcemia. One half of circulating calcium is free (*ionized*) calcium, the only form that has physiologic effects. The remainder is bound to albumin, globulin, and other inorganic molecules. Low albumin levels can affect the total serum calcium level, but the following formula can be used to calculate corrected total serum calcium level:

$$\text{Corrected calcium} = (4.0 - \text{plasma albumin}) \times 0.8\ [\text{serum calcium}]$$

It is important to identify pseudohypercalcemia seen in *hemoconcentration*, paraproteinemia, or thrombocythemia-induced hypercalcemia. Hypercalcemia should be confirmed by repeating total calcium measurements, preferably without venous occlusion. Albumin, phosphate, blood urea nitrogen, and serum creatinine are also measured. Hypophosphatemia is seen in primary hyperparathyroidism and PTH-rp secreting malignancies, but it is not useful in distinguishing these conditions. Normal- or high-serum phosphate, despite correction of dehydration, makes the possibility of a PTH or PTH-rp independent cause of hypercalcemia more likely.

The single most important test helpful in the differential diagnosis of hypercalcemia is the measurement of serum PTH, by a two-site assay specific for the intact, biologically active molecule (iPTH). A low or undetectable serum PTH level, as in our current case study, signifies the presence of non-PTH mediated hypercalcemia that should prompt detailed evaluation for malignancy or other causes of non-PTH mediated hypercalcemia.

A simple algorithm for the evaluation of non-PTH mediated hypercalcemia is shown in figure 6.1.

DISCUSSION

Hypercalcemia is one of the most common and dreaded paraneoplastic complications of malignancy. It occurs in 20% of all patients with cancer. It typically occurs late in the course of malignancy. Often hypercalcemia ushers in the final phase of the disease. The median survival of such hypercalcemia patients is only 30–90 days. Following mechanisms have been uncovered:

1. Elaboration of hypercalcemic factors by solid tumors, termed as humoral hypercalcemia of malignancy (HHM).
2. Severe osteolysis due to bone metastasis.

It is estimated that >80% of malignancy-associated hypercalcemia are HHM. Solid tumors most often associated with hypercalcemia are lung carcinomas (25%), breast carcinomas (20%), squamous cell carcinomas of

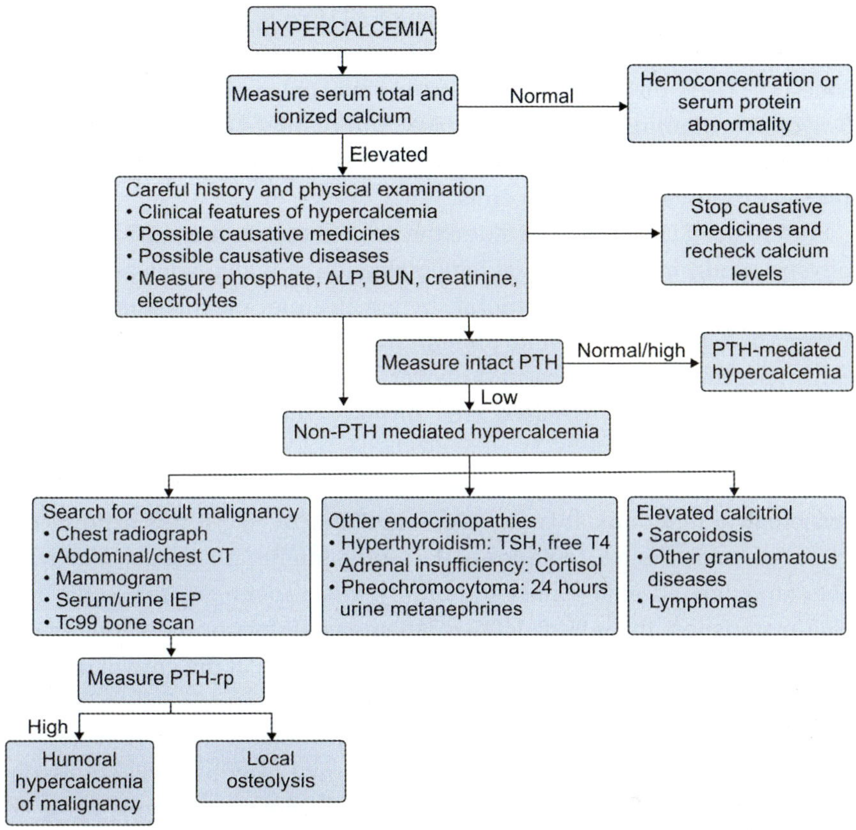

ALP, alkaline phosphatase; BUN, blood urea nitrogen; PTH, parathyroid hormone; TSH, thyroid-stimulating hormone; CT, computed tomography; IEP, immunoelectrophoresis.

Figure 6.1: Evaluation of non-PTH mediated hypercalcemia

head, neck, esophagus or female genital tract (19%), and renal carcinomas (8%). The aggressive T-cell lymphoma associated with human T-cell lymphotropic virus (HTLV-1) infection is the only reported hematological malignancies associated with PTH-rp overproduction and hypercalcemia. A number of factors with bone resorbing activity including PTH, PTH-rp, transforming growth factor α and β, interleukin α and β, epidermal growth factor and prostaglandins have been reported to be responsible for HHM. Among these, parathyroid hormone related peptide (PTH-rp) is the major factor causing HHM.

PTH-like factors responsible for hypercalcemia of malignancy were first proposed by Albright in 1940s. In 1987, PTH-rp was purified from human cancer cells and cloned shortly thereafter. PTH-rp gene encodes a 141 amino acid protein that shares a 60% sequence homology with PTH (over the first 13 amino acids at the amino terminus). Similar to PTH, amino terminal peptides composing the 1–34 sequence of PTH-rp is fully active at the PTH receptor. Thus, PTH-rp would mimic all classic acute effects of PTH. In the kidney, PTH-rp produces phosphaturia, hypocalciuria, and activation of 25-hydroxy vitamin D 1α-hydroxylase, stimulating the synthesis of 1,25 dihydroxy vitamin D. PTH-rp is nearly equipotent with PTH in producing bone resorption and hypercalcemia.

Although PTH-rp and PTH share the same receptor, there are differences between syndromes of humoral hypercalcemia of malignancy and primary hyperparathyroidism. In humoral hypercalcemia of malignancy, bone formation is suppressed, and patients have a metabolic alkalosis rather than hyperchloremic acidosis. Moreover, serum 1,25 dihydroxy vitamin D concentrations are increased in primary hyperparathyroidism and suppressed in cancer.

Apart from its pathological role, PTH-rp also plays a role in some physiological functions. It is not just a mediator of HHM. It is expressed in several normal tissues (epidermis, lactating mammary tissue, pancreatic islets, stomach, adrenal glands and brain). It is also a regulator of placental calcium transport. In the fetus, PTH-rp is responsible for normal endochondral bone formation and controlled cartilage proliferation at the growth plate (its expression in the growth plate is controlled by Indian Hedgehog pathway and its downstream mediator in Gli family, through a negative feedback). PTH-rp has also been to show to regulate normal osteoblast differentiation and activity. PTH-rp is being developed as a potential anabolic agent for osteoporosis treatment.

In a handful of reported cases, malignant tumors secrete PTH and not PTH-rp. Most of these have been lung cancers.

Extensive bone metastasis and local osteolysis accounts for approximately 20% of cases of malignancy-associated hypercalcemia as seen in multiple myeloma and in metastatic breast cancer. Multiple myeloma secretes a host of osteoclast activating factors including macrophage inflammatory protein-1a, receptor activator of nuclear factor kB ligand, interleukin-3, and interleukin-6. In breast cancer, secretion of PTH-rp into the metastatic bone microenvironment further causes pathogenic osteoclast activation and osteolysis.

Vitamin D mediated hypercalcemia can result from intoxication due to inadvertent ingestion of vitamin D. Hypercalcemia in such cases is severe and prolonged due to vitamin D storage in fat. The levels of 25-(OH) vitamin D are dramatically increased. Another mechanism of HHM is overproduction of 1,25-dihydroxy vitamin D in <1% of cases. Hypercalcemia is also associated with granulomatous disorders such as sarcoidosis, tuberculosis, fungal infections, berylliosis, and cancers like

Hodgkin's lymphoma, non-Hodgkin lymphoma, and chronic lymphocytic leukemia, as the macrophages present in these granulomas, and associated malignancies can synthesize calcitriol (1:25 OHD) from 25-(OH) vitamin D. These macrophages express the gene encoding the identical 25-(OH) D 1α-hydroxylase found in the kidney. Acromegaly is another cause for calcitriol-mediated hypercalcemia.

A number of drugs cause hypercalcemia as an adverse effect. Thiazide diuretics exacerbate hypercalcemia due to primary hyperparathyroidism or any other cause. They increase the proximal tubular calcium reabsorption as a result of the direct action of thiazides on the distal tubule. Excess ingestion of vitamin A (retinol) and vitamin A derivatives like isotretinoin and tretinoin can occasionally cause hypercalcemia due to stimulation of bone resorption. The triad of hypercalcemia, metabolic alkalosis, and renal failure called the milk alkali syndrome (Burnett's syndrome) is the consequence of massive ingestion of calcium and absorbable alkali.

Some other endocrinopathies apart from hyperparathyroidism are also known to cause hypercalcemia. Hyperthyroidism mildly raises serum calcium levels by increasing bone resorption. Adrenal insufficiency causes hypercalcemia by causing volume contraction and increased albumin levels. Pheochromocytoma causes hypercalcemia through PTH-rp production.

Williams' syndrome: A developmental disorder with random genetic mutation (deletion of small piece of chromosome 7) with supravalvular aortic stenosis, elfin facies, and mental retardation is associated with transient hypercalcemia in the first 4 years of life. Additional features include star like pattern of iris, and risk of prediabetes, diabetes mellitus.

Jansen's metaphyseal-chondrodysplasia (ligand independent activation of PTH-type 1 receptor) is another rare genetic disease in which affected persons present in childhood with short stature, micrognathia, hypercalcemia, and hypophosphatemia.

Immobilization due to spinal cord injury or extensive casting after fractures can lead to bone resorption sufficient to cause hypercalcemia. Hypercalcemia also occurs in other conditions of high bone turnover such as Paget's disease.

MANAGEMENT

Differentiating between various etiologies of hypercalcemia has prognostic significance. Primary hyperparathyroidism is a benign, treatable disease with a likelihood of survival past 100 days. On the other hand, an elevated PTH-rp driven hypercalcemia of malignancy is associated with a high mortality within 100 days.

Aggressive management of acute severe hypercalcemia in malignancy can reverse patient's symptoms for several weeks and can provide opportunity for treatment underlying tumor, if it is treatable. Only effective treatment of the underlying neoplasm can significantly influence the long-term prognosis for patients with malignant hypercalcemia.

Treatment of serum calcium concentrations <12 mg/dL aims solely at the treatment of the underlying disorder. Urgent interventions are needed in case of presence of symptoms and signs of hypercalcemia and serum calcium concentrations exceeding 12 mg/dL. Calcium concentration >14 mg/dL almost always needs aggressive management.

The first priority is to correct extracellular volume depletion, which is invariably present, by infusing isotonic saline at the rate of 2–4 L in 24–48 hours. Hydration enhances urinary calcium excretion by increasing the glomerular filtration of calcium and decreasing tubular reabsorption of sodium and calcium (solvent drag). This form of therapy should, however, be used cautiously in patients with compromised cardiovascular and renal function. After hydration has been achieved small doses of loop diuretics may be added to promote calciuresis.

Since accelerated bone resorption is an important factor contributing to acute hypercalcemia, next line of measures involve use of antiresorptive agents, bisphosphonates being the agents of choice. The US Food and Drug Administration have approved intravenous Pamidronate and Zoledronate for treatment of malignant hypercalcemia.

Serum calcium usually declines within 24 hours and reaches a nadir within 1 week after a single infusion. These drugs generally are well tolerated, although local pain or swelling at the infusion site, low-grade fever lasting 1–2 days after the infusion, transient lymphopenia, and mild hypophosphatemia or hypomagnesemia may occur. Intravenous bisphosphonates can be nephrotoxic. Calcitonin is a peptide hormone, which is a safe therapeutic agent for a more rapid control of hypercalcemia. Calcitonin inhibits osteoclast-mediated resorption and also increases renal calcium excretion. It has a rapid onset of action, causing serum calcium to fall by 2 mg/dL within 2–6 hours of administration. Unfortunately, this agent is not as potent as the most potent bisphosphonates and tachyphylaxis may occur after 24–48 hours.

Intravenous or oral glucocorticoids are considered in patients with suspected vitamin D-dependent hypercalcemia, including those with lymphoma or granulomatous disease. The response to glucocorticoids is more delayed than that of bisphosphonates.

Whereas severe renal insufficiency precludes saline rehydration or use of bisphosphonates, dialysis against a low or zero calcium dialysate would be most appropriate. After correcting acute severe hypercalcemia, attention should be directed to treatment of the underlying disease causing hypercalcemia.

KEY POINTS

- Hypercalcemia is most commonly caused by cancer or parathyroid disease
- Patients with mild-to-moderate hypercalcemia are typically asymptomatic and hypercalcemia is often diagnosed on routine blood work
- Incidentally diagnosed hypercalcemia is most likely due to an abnormality in the parathyroid
- Hypercalcemia of malignancy seldom has a subtle presentation
- When symptoms present, they can be of gastrointestinal, renal, or psychiatric manifestation
- The first step in assessing the etiology of hypercalcemia is to determine whether the hypercalcemia is PTH dependent or not
- General measures for correcting hypercalcemia include volume repletion, loop diuretics, such as furosemide, enabling an increase in the urinary excretion of calcium following rehydration. Antiresorptive, such as calcitonin and bisphosphonates, can decrease further bone resorption
- Definitive treatment of hypercalcemia can only be completed once the causative mechanism is identified.

SUGGESTED READINGS

1. Donovan PJ, Sundac L, Pretorious CJ, et al. Calcitriol-mediated hypercalcemia: causes and course in 101 patients. J Clin Endocrinol Metab. 2013;98:4023-9.
2. Jacobs TP, Bilezikian JP. Clinical reviews: rare causes of hypercalcemia. J Clin Endocrinol Metab. 2005; 90:316-22.
3. Mudd AH, van den Berg H, Boshuis PG, et al. Ectopic production of 1:25-dihydroxyvitamin D by B-cell lymphoma as a cause of hypercalcemia. Cancer. 1987;59:1543-6.
4. Patel AM, Adeseun GA, Goldfarb S. Calcium-Alkali Syndrome in modern era. Nutrients. 2013;5:488-93.
5. Sharma OP. Hypercalcemia in granulomatous disorders: a clinical review. Curr Opin Pulm Med. 2000; 6:442-7.
6. Suva LJ, Winslow GA, Wettenhall RE, et al. A parathyroid hormone-related protein implicated in malignant hypercalcemia: cloning and expression. Science. 1987;237:893-6.

CHAPTER

7

Secondary Hyperparathyroidism

Shruti Sharma, Naresh Bansal, Surya K Singh

INTRODUCTION

We present two interesting cases of secondary hyperparathyroidism (SHPT) with metabolic bone disease due to vitamin D deficiency. Low socioeconomic status, poor dietary intake, inadequate sunlight exposure, dark skin, and prolonged breastfeeding contributed to nutritional osteomalacia in our first case. Other causes of osteomalacia including malabsorbtive states and renal tubular disorders were ruled out before diagnosing nutritional cause. This patient showed characteristic skeletal feature that improved up on receiving vitamin D replacement and calcium supplementation. Our second case had chronic kidney disease (CKD)—metabolic bone disease.

Chronic renal insufficiency is the most common cause of hyperparathyroidism. Increased parathyroid hormone (PTH) (>600 pg/mL) was found to be an independent risk factor for all-cause and cardiovascular mortality in dialysis outcomes and practice patterns study. Serum levels of calcium, phosphorus, and intact PTH should be measured in all patients with CKD with estimated glomerular filtration rate (GFR) <60 mL/min. The normalization of serum calcium and phosphorus with suppression of PTH values should be the goal of treatment.

Metabolic bone disease should always be suspected in case of bony deformities in children or bone pains proximal weakness, severe osteopenia, or fragility fractures in adults. Investigations should include biochemical tests and radiological imaging for etiological diagnosis. Serum PTH assay is helpful in diagnosing SHPT, monitoring, and prognosis of such cases.

CASE PRESENTATION

Case 1

A 37-year-old lady with no formal school education and low socioeconomic status presented with complaints of severe bone pains and bony deformities of 1 year duration with difficulty in rising from a chair and walking. There was no history of diarrhea, jaundice, or urinary complaints or any previous drug intake. She had an insufficient intake of milk and milk products with poor sunlight exposure and history of obstructed labor with prolonged breastfeeding of two children for 16–18 months.

On physical examination her height, weight, and BMI were 144 cm, 31 kg, and 15 kg/m^2, respectively. Pallor was present. She had 4/5th power in shoulder and pelvic girdle muscles with waddling gait. Other systemic examinations were normal.

Laboratory tests showed microcytic hypochromic type anemia with hemoglobin of 8.0 g/dL. The corrected serum calcium was 8.19 mg/dL, serum phosphorus 2.3 mg/dL, and serum alkaline phosphatase 796 IU/L. Other laboratory data were normal including erythrocyte sedimentation rate, serum creatine kinase, liver enzymes, and renal function tests. Further work-up revealed low 25-hydroxy vitamin D [6.4 ng/mL (normal: 30–60 ng/mL)], and high iPTH [236 pg/mL (normal: 8–80 pg/mL)]. The 24-hour urinary calcium was 40 mg/day. Anti-tTG (tissue transglutaminase) antibodies were negative and thyroid function tests were normal. Skeletal survey revealed generalized osteoporosis and pseudofractures of tibia (Figs 7.1 and 7.2).

The diagnosis of osteomalacia was made based on clinical, biochemical, and radiological features. She was treated with calcium and high-dose vitamin D 600,000 IU intramuscularly that led to dramatic clinical improvement.

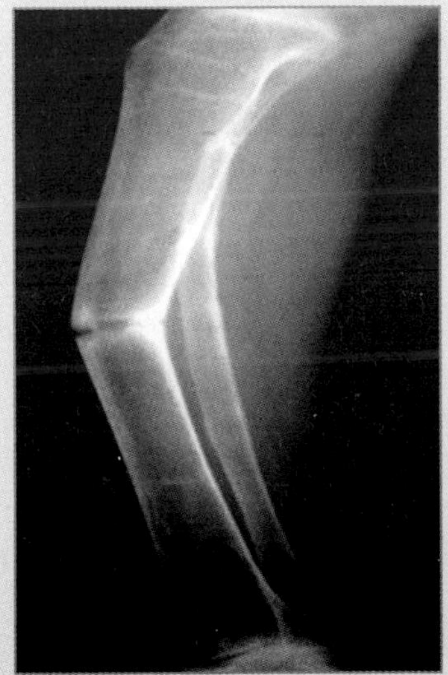

Figure 7.1: Pseudofracture of the left tibia

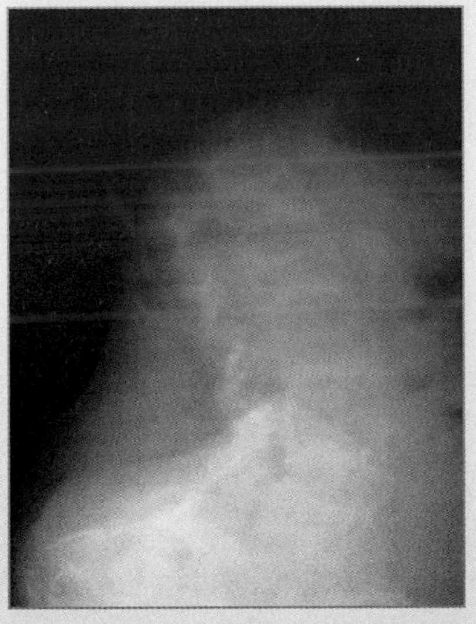

Figure 7.2: Generalized osteoporosis with codfish vertebra

Case 2

A 45-year-old woman presented with complaints of swelling over the legs for 5 months, breathlessness on exertion for 3 months, low backache, and bone pains for 3 months and decrease in urine output for 1 month. There was no history of diabetes, hypertension, jaundice, chest pain, palpitations, jaundice, or abdominal distention.

On physical examination, her BMI was 19.3 kg/m^2. Pallor and pedal edema were present. Pulse was 88/minute. BP was 170/100 mmHg in right upper limb. Systemic examinations were normal.

Laboratory tests revealed microcytic anemia (hemoglobin of 8 g/dL and mean corpuscular volume of 72 fL). Serum creatinine/urea was 4.8/94 mg/dL. The corrected serum calcium/phosphorus/ alkaline phosphatase were 8.8 mg/dL/ 5.8 mg/dL/400 IU/L, respectively. Serum sodium/potassium were 135/5.5 mEq/L. Urine examination showed 2+ albumin 0.25(OH) D was 16 ng/mL and iPTH was 800 pg/mL. Collagen profile and complement levels were normal.

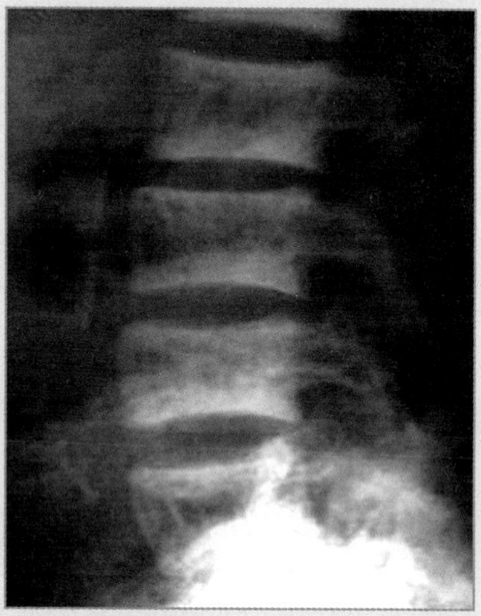

Figure 7.3: Rugger jersy spine

Skeletal survey (Fig. 7.3) showed generalized osteopenia with diffuse sclerosis of vertebral endplates "rugger jersy spine." In USG of abdomen, small-sized kidneys (left kidney: 6.2 cm, right kidney: 6.0 cm) with increased echogenicity were present.

Patient was diagnosed with CKD. She was advised renal replacement therapy. Phosphorus binder calcium acetate and calcitriol were given along with antihypertensive, hematinic, and erythropoietin injection.

DISCUSSION

Unlike primary hyperparathyroidism, where high levels of PTH are autonomously produced by the parathyroid glands, SHPT refers to high PTH levels caused by conditions like hypocalcemia, hyperphosphatemia, or hypovitaminosis D that directly stimulate parathyroid glands to increase the synthesis of PTH. Chronic renal insufficiency is the most common cause of SHPT worldwide. It has been demonstrated that the PTH levels start to increase as early as the beginning of CKD stage III (estimated GFR <60 mL/min), along with normal levels of serum calcium and phosphorus in CKD patients. Other common causes are insufficient calcium intake, decreased intestinal calcium absorption, insufficient vitamin D intake, and malabsorption.

Vitamin D deficiency causes rickets in children and osteomalacia in adults. The cause of vitamin D deficiency can be a result of deficient production of vitamin D in the skin especially in dark-skinned individual, lack of dietary intake, intestinal malabsorption, accelerated loss of vitamin D by drugs (antiseizure medications), or hepatic disease and impaired 1α-hydroxylation due to renal disease. Mutation in 1α-hydroxylase or resistance to the biologic effects of $1{,}25(OH)_2$ D are causes of hereditary vitamin D resistant rickets. Long-standing vitamin D deficiency results in hypocalcemia that stimulates PTH production in parathyroid glands resulting in SHPT, impaired mineralization of the skeleton with appearance of looser zones or pseudo fractures (Fig. 7.1) and proximal myopathy. Vitamin D deficiency also has been shown to be associated with an increase in overall mortality rates, including cardiovascular causes. Treatment is 60,000 IU of oral vitamin D3 weekly for 3–12 weeks followed by maintenance therapy (800 IU daily) or vitamin D3 2–10,000 IU daily for 4–6 weeks single oral (or IM) vitamin D3 of 600,000 units (Stoss Therapy) is also recommended. Vitamin D should always be replenished in conjunction with calcium supplementation in the form of 1.5–2 g of daily elemental calcium. In patients in whom 1α-hydroxylation is impaired active $1{,}25(OH)_2$ D3 (calcitriol) is given in doses of 0.25–0.5 µg/day. Monitoring is done by serum and urinary calcium measurements. In patients who are vitamin D replete and are taking adequate calcium supplementation, the 24-hour urinary calcium excretion should be in the range of 100–250 mg/24 hours.

Renal osteodystrophy is bone disease associated with SHPT. It is part of a spectrum of mineral metabolism; vascular and skeletal complications are seen in the syndrome of chronic kidney disease–mineral bone disorder (CKD–MBD). Renal osteodystrophy is classified as osteitis fibrosa, osteomalacia, or mixed, mild, or adynamic disease, according to the histologic features. The classic histologic form of renal osteodystrophy is osteitis fibrosa, which is caused by SHPT. Declining renal function leads to decreased renal phosphate excretion, increased serum phosphorous, elevated levels of fibroblast growth factor 23 (FGF-23), and reduced synthesis of calcitriol. These changes result in increased synthesis and secretion of PTH and parathyroid hyperplasia, contributing to the development of a vicious cycle. Raised PTH causes increased bone remodeling and resorption of bone.

In children SHPT may present as growth retardation and skeletal deformities, whereas in adult bone pain muscle weakness or fractures may occur. Extraskeletal soft tissue calcification and vascular calcifications are also present. Aortic calcifications, mitral annular calcinosis, and coronary artery disease are common and an independent predictive factor of increased vascular morbidity and mortality.

Biochemical abnormalities include hyperphosphatemia, decreased 1,25 dihydroxy vitamin D levels, and raised PTH levels. Radiological finding shows generalized osteopenia with subperiosteal resorption commonly seen on the radial aspect of the middle phalanges, acro-osteolysis may be visible at the finger tips, the lateral end of the clavicle and the calcaneus. Alterations on X-rays of the skull include diminished or increased bone density, radiolucent areas, described as "pepper pot skull." The widespread and diffuse sclerosis of bone occurs and is most prominent in the vertebral endplates, giving "rugger jersey spine" appearance (Fig. 7.3).

The treatment of SHPT in patients with CKD involves the use of phosphate binders, active vitamin D analog, and calcimimetic. Early suppression of PTH secretion may prevent subsequent parathyroid gland hyperplasia. As dialysis patients are relatively resistant to the actions of PTH, a PTH level within the normal range is not useful and different PTH goals are recommended for various levels of CKD PTH target values are 35–70, 70–110, and 150–300 pg/mL for CKD stage III, IV, V, respectively. Failure of medical therapy to control hyperparathyroidism (iPTH levels of ≥400–500 pg/mL persist), severe bone pain or fracture, pruritus, and calciphylaxis are indications for surgery. Figure 7.4 gives an overview of approach to a case of metabolic bone disease that may help clinician to plan the relevant investigations.

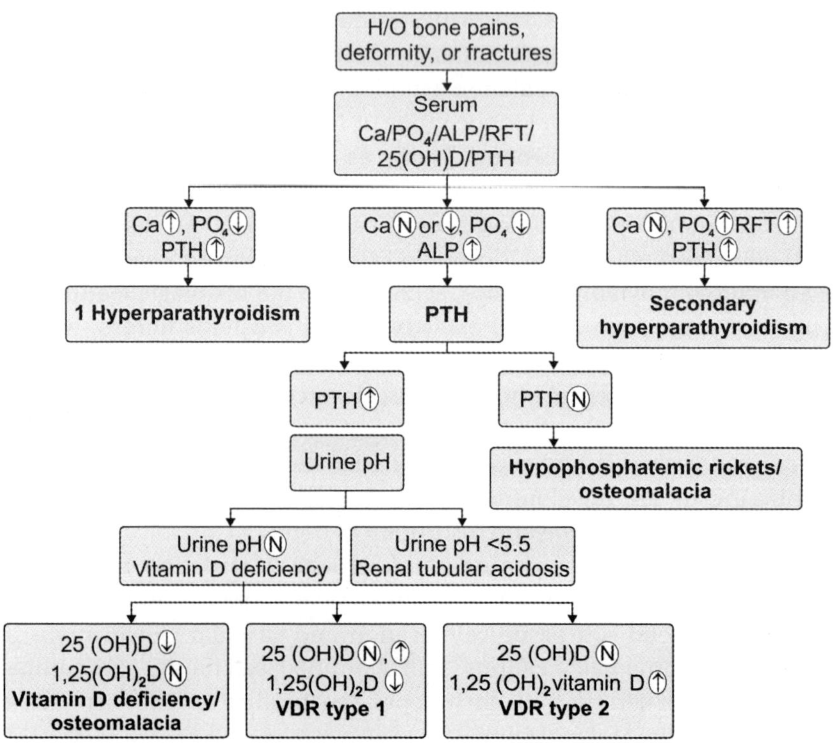

Ca, calcium; PO_4, phosphate; PTH, parathyroid hormone; ALP, alkaline phosphatase; RFT, renal function test; VDR, vitamin D receptor; 25(OH)vitamin D, 25-hydroxy vitamin D; $25(OH)_2$vitamin D, 25-dihydroxy vitamin D; ⓓ, Decrease; ⓘ, Increase; Ⓝ, Normal.

Figure 7.4: An approach to a case of metabolic bone disease

KEY POINTS

- Chronic kidney disease is the most common cause of hyperparathyroidism, followed by vitamin D deficiency
- Serum intact parathyroid hormone (PTH) is useful in diagnosing and monitoring SHPT
- The goal of treatment is normalization of serum calcium and phosphorus with suppression of PTH.

SUGGESTED READINGS

1. Holick MF. Vitamin D deficiency. N Engl J Med. 2007;357:266.
2. K/DOQI clinical practice guidelines for bone metabolism and disease in chronic kidney disease. Am J Kidney Dis. 2003;42(Suppl. 3):S1.
3. Pettifor JM. Rickets and vitamin D deficiency in children and adoles-cents. Endocrinol Metab Clin North Am. 2005; 34:537-53.
4. Pitts TO, Piraino BH, Mitro R, et al. Hyperparathyroidism and 1,25-dihydroxyvitamin D deficiency in mild, moderate, and severe renal failure. J Clin Endocrinol Metab. 1988;67:876.
5. Tentori F, Blayney MJ, Albert JM, et al. Mortality risk for dialysis patients with different levels of serum calcium, phosphorus, and PTH: the Dialysis Outcomes and Practice Patterns Study (DOPPS). Am J Kidney Dis. 2008;52:519-30.

CHAPTER

8

Juvenile Hypothyroidism Presenting as Precocious Puberty

Sarita Bajaj

CASE PRESENTATION

A five-year girl was brought by her parents for continuous vaginal bleeding of 15-days duration. There was no history of systemic or central nervous system disease, febrile illness, drug intake, maternal disease, or medication during pregnancy. Milestones were delayed for the last 2 years. Her performance in preschool had deteriorated.

Her face was puffy and dull looking with coarse facial features and normal dentition. Skin was dry and rough. Breasts tanner stage 3 with no axillary or pubic hair. The thyroid gland was normal on examination. She weighed 15 kg and was 89.5 cm tall (<25th percentile).

Hormone profile confirmed primary hypothyroidism with hyperprolactinemia.

INVESTIGATIONS

- Free T3: 0.5 pg/mL (normal: 1.4–4.4 pg/mL)
- Free T4: Undetectable (normal: 0.8–2 ng/mL)
- Thyroid-stimulating hormone (TSH): >100 uIU/mL (normal: 0.2–5 uIU/mL)
- Prolactin: 135 ng/mL (normal: 0–20 ng/mL)
- Luteinizing hormone (LH): 0.4 mIU/mL (normal: 1.8–13 mIU/mL)
- Follicle-stimulating hormone (FSH): 2.5 mIU/mL (normal: 2–10 mIU/mL)
- Estradiol: 10.5 pg/mL (normal: 30–120 pg/mL).

No evidence of fibrous dysplasia or café-au-lait spots. Bone age was 3 years 6 months (Greulich Pyle method). Ultrasound of pelvis showed a bulky uterus with cysts in the left ovary. An enhanced computed tomography of the cranium was normal.

She was started with replacement dose of levothyroxine that resulted in cessation of vaginal bleeding and correction of all associated features within 3 months.

DISCUSSION

Sexual precocity may be considered as the appearance of any sign of secondary sexual maturation below the normal onset of puberty: 9 years for boys, 7 years for Caucasian girls, and 6 years for African-American girls.

Patient was diagnosed as hypothyroid with incomplete GnRH-independent isosexual precocious puberty in view of the breast development and menstruation in the absence of pubic or axillary hair with normal gonadotropin levels.

Gonadotropin-independent precocious puberty (GIPP) (also known as peripheral precocious puberty or pseudoprecocious puberty) is caused by excess secretion of sex hormones (estrogens or androgens) derived either from the gonads or adrenal glands or from exogenous sources. Further characterization is based upon whether the sexual characteristics are appropriate for the child's gender (isosexual) or inappropriate, with virilization of girls and feminization of boys (contrasexual). FSH and LH levels are suppressed (in the prepubertal range) and do not increase with GnRH stimulation.

Differential Diagnosis of Incomplete GnRH-Independent Isosexual Precocious Puberty in a Female (Table 8.1)

1. *Ovarian cysts*: A large functioning follicular cyst of the ovaries is the most common cause of GIPP in girls. Affected patients often present after an episode of vaginal bleeding. These cysts may appear and regress spontaneously; conservative management is usually appropriate. Ovarian cysts are often seen in adolescent girls and young women who become hypothyroid. Cysts may also be seen in those attempting weight loss through severe caloric restriction.
2. *Ovarian tumors*: Ovarian tumors are a rare cause of GIPP in girls. Granulosa cell tumors may cause isosexual GIPP. Sertoli/Leydig cell tumors (arrhenoblastoma), pure Leydig cell tumors, and gonadoblastoma may make androgens and cause contrasexual GIPP.
3. Adrenal estrogen-secreting tumors: It may lead to feminization. Rarely, adrenal tumors can produce androgen and estrogen, the latter because of intra-adrenal aromatization of androgen (or enough androgen that is peripherally aromatized to estrogen), causing both male and female pubertal changes.

TABLE 8.1: Classification of precocious puberty in females
Central (complete or true) GnRH-dependent isosexual precocious puberty
• Constitutional
• Idiopathic
• Central nervous system disorders (including congenital defects)
• Tumors
• Infection
• Trauma
• Radiation
• Following androgen exposure
Incomplete GnRH-independent isosexual precocious puberty
• Ovarian cysts
• Estrogen-secreting neoplasms
• Peutz–Jeghers syndrome
• McCune–Albright syndrome
• Hypothyroidism
• Iatrogenic or exogenous sexual precocity
Incomplete contrasexual precocity
• Androgen-secreting tumor
• Virilizing congenital adrenal hyperplasia
• Iatrogenic sexual precocity due to gonadotropin or sex steroid exposure
• Variation in pubertal development
• Premature thelarche
• Premature menarche
• Premature pubarche

4. *McCune-Albright syndrome* (MAS): McCune–Albright syndrome, a rare disorder characterized by the triad of peripheral precocious puberty, café-au-lait spots, and fibrous dysplasia of bone. McCune–Albright syndrome should be considered in girls with recurrent formation of follicular cysts and cyclic menses. Cutaneous manifestations and bone lesions may increase over time. In girls presenting with vaginal bleeding, the ovarian enlargement has often been mistaken for an ovarian tumor, leading to mistaken oophorectomy. Girls presenting with premature vaginal bleeding need to be carefully evaluated for features of MAS to avoid this mistake. The clinical phenotype is markedly variable, but precocious puberty is the most common manifestation. As in other forms of GIPP, the sequence of pubertal progression may be abnormal, in that vaginal bleeding often precedes significant breast development. Prolonged exposure to elevated levels of sex steroids may cause accelerated growth,

advanced skeletal maturation, and compromised adult height. Although the precocious puberty is typically GIPP, a secondary component of gonadotropin-dependent precocious puberty may develop, also because of prolonged exposure to sex steroids.

5. *Exogenous estrogen*: Feminization has been attributed to excess estrogen exposure from proprietary creams, ointments, sprays, food contamination, and alternative remedies. Prescribing topical estrogens to treat menopausal symptoms may inadvertently expose children to the hormones.
6. *Peutz-Jeghers syndrome*: Fallopian mucinous tumors; unique ovarian sex cord tumors with annular tubules that cause heavy menstrual periods and lead to isosexual precocity; testicular sex cord and Sertoli cell tumors, leading to sexual precocity and gynecomastia in boys.

Hypothyroidism in prepubertal years usually leads to short stature and may lead to delay in sexual maturation. Hypothyroidism is indeed the most common endocrine cause for short stature. Rarely incomplete isosexual precocity may occur. Girls may have breast development, enlarged labia minora, and estrogenic change in the vaginal smear though without the appearance of pubic hair. Some girls have severe vaginal bleeding with solitary or multiple functional ovarian cysts being demonstrable by pelvic sonography. Therapy with levothyroxine results in reversal of all these features. Growth obtundation is the most significant sign and associated bone age retardation is dependent on the duration of thyroid deficiency. Mental functions are usually normal; mental retardation is usually not seen in children with onset of hypothyroidism after the age of 3 years. Scholastic performance may or may not be affected.

Several hypotheses have been proposed to explain this disorder:

- TRH action on the gonadotrophs (apart from the thyrotrophs) and TSH action on the gonad via FSH receptor (specificity spill over)
- Hyperprolactinemia as a result of chronic TRH stimulation of the pituitary possibly plays an important role in causing sexual precocity by sensitizing the ovaries to the low circulating levels of gonadotropins.
- Alteration in metabolism of gonadal steroids.

There may be an overlap in the pituitary production of TSH and gonadotrophs with the latter causing early ovarian secretion of estrogen and subsequent endometrial stimulation with vaginal bleeding. In the presence of an elevated prolactin, galactorrhea may be demonstrable. Because there is no pubertal increase in the adrenal production of androgen precursors, axillary, and pubic hair are not apparent.

THYROID DISEASE IN CHILDHOOD AND ADOLESCENCE

Hypothyroidism in the pediatric age group is quite challenging and not infrequent (as many as 3% of the population may be affected). Acquired hypothyroidism is not associated with permanent effects on cognition, but affected individuals may have permanent short stature, particularly in severe hypothyroidism. The long-term impact of subclinical hypothyroidism in infancy childhood and adolescence is unclear. Treatment, however, with L-thyroxine is relatively safe and inexpensive.

Chronic Lymphocytic Thyroiditis

The most frequent cause of hypothyroidism in children and adolescents is chronic lymphocytic thyroiditis (CLT), an autoimmune disease which is closely related to Graves' disease. Both goitrous (Hashimoto's disease) and nongoitrous (primary hypothyroidism) variants of thyroiditis have been identified. It has a striking predilection for females with a family history of autoimmune thyroid disease (both CLT and Graves' disease) (found in 30–40% of subjects). Adolescence is the most common age at presentation during childhood, but it can be seen at any age after the neonatal period, even in infants six months of age. Antibodies to thyroglobulin (Tg) and thyroid peroxidase (TPO-more sensitive) are detectable in a majority of patients with CLT and serve as useful markers of underlying autoimmunity.

Goiter (mostly euthyroid) may be present in approximately two thirds of children with CLT. Although hypothyroidism is the most common functional abnormality, patients may occasionally be hyperthyroid.

Thyroid Dysgenesis and Inborn Errors of Thyroid Hormonogenesis

Occasionally patients with mild thyroid dysgenesis will escape detection by new-born screening and present later in childhood with nongoitrous hypothyroidism or with an enlarging mass at the base of the tongue or along the course of the thyroglossal duct. Similarly children with milder inborn errors of thyroid hormonogenesis may only be recognized later in childhood because of the detection of a goiter.

Iodine and Other Micronutrient Deficiency: Natural Goitrogens

In areas of endemic iodine deficiency hypothyroidism may be aggravated by the coincident ingestion of goitrogen containing foods such as cassava, soybeans, broccoli, cabbage, sweet potatoes, and cauliflower or by certain water pollutants. Iodine deficiency may also be exacerbated by lack of selenium a component of the selenocysteine thyroid hormone deiodinases.

CLINICAL MANIFESTATIONS

The onset of hypothyroidism in childhood is insidious. Affected children are recognized either because of the detection of a goiter on routine examination or because of poor growth sometimes for several years prior to diagnosis. Because, linear growth tends to be more affected than weight, patients therefore, are relatively overweight for their height, but rarely obese. Dental and skeletal maturation are significantly delayed. Van Wyk and Grumbach syndrome is interesting in that it is the only entity associated with precocious puberty where the bone age is delayed.

The classical clinical manifestations of hypothyroidism may be present, but are often not the presenting complaints. School performance is not usually affected. A delayed relaxation of the deep tendon reflexes may be elicited in severe cases. The thyroid gland in CLT is diffusely enlarged and has a rubbery consistency. If asymmetric, it must be distinguished from thyroid neoplasia.

The absence of goiter suggests the diagnosis of primary hypothyroidism, thyroid dysgenesis or secondary/tertiary hypothyroidism (Table 8.2 and Fig. 8.1).

TABLE 8.2: Causes of hypothyroidism in childhood and adolescence
Primary hypothyroidism
• Chronic lymphocytic thyroiditis
• Iodine deficiency/goitrogens
• Drugs
• Miscellaneous
○ Mantle irradiation
○ Cystinosis
○ Histiocytosis X
○ Mitochondrial disease
○ Hemangiomas ("consumptive hypothyroidism")
Secondary or tertiary hypothyroidism
• Brain irradiation/surgery
• Brain tumor (craniopharyngioma)
• Congenital hypopituitarism
Abnormal thyroid hormone action
• Thyroid hormone resistance (TRβ mutation)
• Abnormal T4 transport monocarboxylate transporter 8 MCT8) mutation)

Source: Cooper D. Medical Management of Thyroid Disease, 2nd edition. 2008. p. 347.

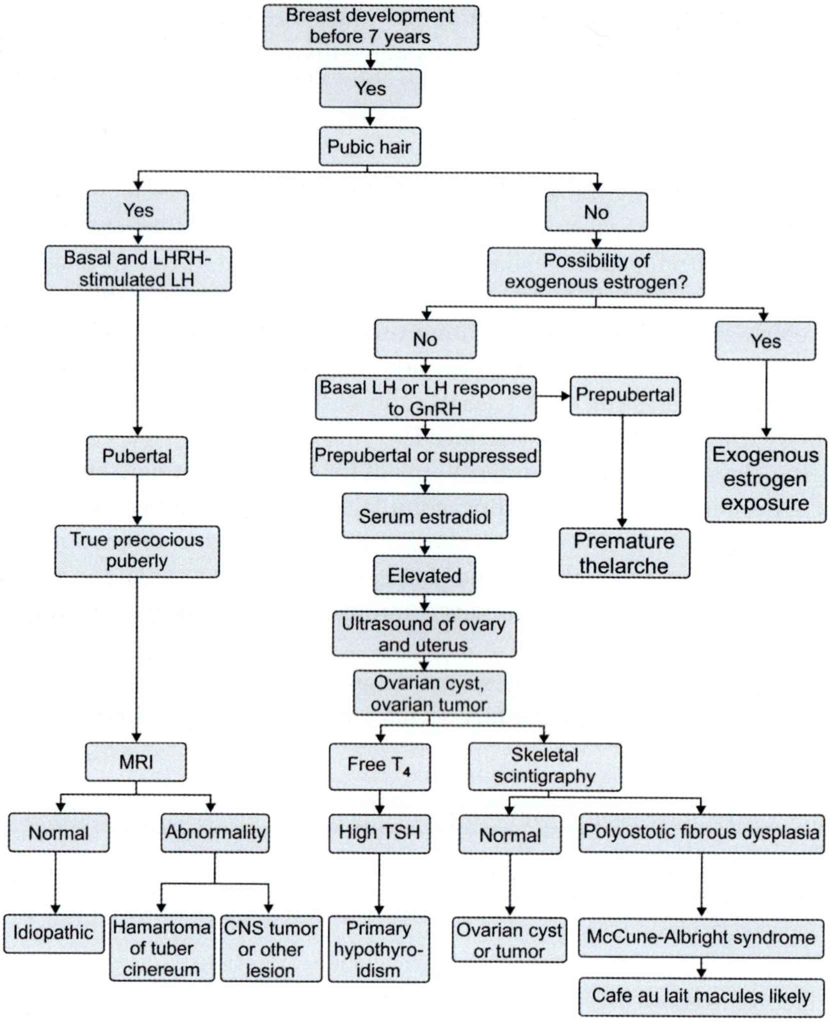

LHRH, luteinizing-hormone-releasing hormone; LH, luteinizing hormone; MRI, magnetic resonance imaging; TSH, thyroid-stimulating hormone; CNS, central nervous system; GnRH, gonadotropin-releasing hormone.

Figure 8.1: Approach to a case of isosexual precocity in a female

Puberty tends to be delayed in hypothyroid children although sexual precocity has been described in long-standing severe hypothyroidism. Females may menstruate but commonly have breast development with little sexual hair. Ovarian cysts may be demonstrated on ultrasonography; galactorrhea due to hyperprolactinemia may also be seen. The incidence of slipped femoral capital epiphyses is increased in hypothyroid children. The sella turcica may be enlarged due to thyrotroph hyperplasia in patients with long-standing and severe hypothyroidism. This is reversible with thyroid hormone replacement.

LABORATORY EVALUATION

Measurement of TSH is the best initial screening test for the presence of primary hypothyroidism. If the TSH is elevated, measurement of free T4 will distinguish whether the child has compensated (normal free T4) or overt (low free T4) hypothyroidism. Measurement of free hormones must be avoided during protein fluxes such as seen during acute sickness. Presence of antibodies will interfere with free hormone measurements.

Measurement of TSH is not helpful in secondary or tertiary hypothyroidism. Hypothyroidism in these cases is demonstrated by the presence of a low free T4 with an inappropriately low or normal TSH. Occasionally mild TSH elevation is seen in individuals with hypothalamic hypothyroidism a consequence of the secretion of a TSH molecule with impaired bioactivity but normal immunoreactivity. Thyroid hormone resistance is characterized by elevated levels of free T4 and T3 and an inappropriately normal or elevated TSH concentration.

Chronic lymphocytic thyroiditis is diagnosed by elevated titers of Tg and/or TPO Abs. Ancillary investigations (thyroid ultrasonography and/or thyroid scintigraphy) may be performed if thyroid Ab tests are negative or if a nodule is palpable. If thyroid Ab tests are negative and no goiter is present thyroid ultrasonography and/or scan identify the presence and location of thyroid tissue and thereby distinguish primary hypothyroidism from thyroid dysgenesis.

TREATMENT OF ACQUIRED HYPOTHYROIDISM IN CHILDREN

In acquired hypothyroidism, rapid replacement is not essential in children >3 years of age in whom brain development is not the primary concern. This is particularly true in children with long-standing, severe thyroid underactivity in whom rapid normalization may result in undesirable side effects (deterioration in scholastic performance, short attention span, hyperactivity, insomnia, and behavioral problems). In these children it is preferable to increase the replacement dose slowly over several weeks to months. Severely hypothyroid children should also be observed closely for complaints of severe headache when therapy is initiated, because of the rare development of pseudotumor cerebri or psychosis. In contrast full replacement can be initiated at once without risk of adverse events in children with mild hypothyroidism.

The replacement dose of L-thyroxine in childhood is approximately 100 μg/m^2 or 4–6 μg/kg for children 1–5 years of age, 3–4 μg/kg for those ages

6–10 years, and 2–3 μg/kg for those 11 years of age and older. In patients with a goiter, a somewhat higher L-thyroxine dosage is used to keep the TSH in the low normal range (0.3–1.0 mU/L in an ultrasensitive assay), and thereby minimize its goitrogenic effects. Serum T4/free T4 and TSH concentration should be measured after the child has received the recommended dosage for at least 6–8 weeks, preferably at the same time of day. Once a euthyroid state has been achieved patients should be monitored every 6–12 months and 6–8 weeks after any dosage change. Interval growth as well as maintenance of a euthyroid state is closely monitored. Thyroid hormone replacement is usually not associated with weight loss in overweight children except in severe hypothyroidism. Some children with severe, long-standing hypothyroidism at diagnosis do not achieve their adult height potential even with apparently optimal therapy emphasizing the importance of early diagnosis and treatment. Osteoporosis is another potential complication of overtreatment. Therapy is continued lifelong.

KEY POINTS

- In a child presenting with precocious puberty and delayed bone age, hypothyroidism must be excluded
- Treatment of hypothyroidism leads to rapid normalization of both biochemical as well as clinical features
- In those with pituitary enlargement, neurosurgical intervention is often unnecessary since thyrotroph hyperplasia will dissipate following appropriate thyroid hormone replacement.

SUGGESTED READINGS

1. Bruder JM, Samuels MH, Bremner WJ, et al. Hypothyroidism-induced macro-orchidism use of a gonadotropin-releasing hormone agonist to understand its mechanism and augment adult stature. J Clin Endocrinol Metab. 1995;80:11-6.
2. Cooper D. Medical Management of Thyroid Disease, 2nd edition. 2008.
3. Gardner DG, Shoback D. Acute adrenal insufficiency. In: Basic and Clinical Endocrinology, 9th edition. Greenspan's: McGraw Hill; 2011. p. 238.
4. Gordon CM, Austin DJ, Radovick S, et al. Primary hypothyroidism presenting as severe vaginal bleeding in a prepubertal girl. J Pediatr Adolesc Gyneol. 1997;10(1):35-8.
5. Styn DM, Grumbach MM. Puberty: ontogeny, neuroendocrinology, physiology and disorders. In: Kronenberg HM, Melmed S, (eds). William's Textbook of Endocrinology, 11th edition. Philadelphia, USA: Elsevier Inc; 2008.
6. Van Wyk JJ, Grumbach MM. syndrome of precocious menstruation and galactorrhea in juvenile hypothyroidism an example of hormonal overlap in pituitary feedback. J Pediatr. 1960;57:416-35.

CHAPTER

9

Hypopituitarism: Sheehan's Syndrome

RV Jayakumar

CASE PRESENTATION

A 44-year-old lady presented for second opinion regarding abnormal thyroid function tests. She has complaints of tiredness and weakness for last 10 months, which is slowly progressive. There is no history suggestive of underlying infectious etiology. She has noticed slight decrease in appetite and has lost weight (2 kg) during last 6 months. She used to have vague abdominal pain on and off for which no attention was sought. Her bowel habits are normal. She has no specific muscle weakness like difficulty in getting up from squatting position or combing hair, but generally feels weakness after doing small household chores that she performed in the past without any difficulty. She denies headache or vomiting, but occasionally feels nauseated. During an episode of flu, which all her family members had contracted, she was found to be extremely weak and was taken to an emergency unit of a nearby hospital. She was seen by a physician who noted pallor and her symptoms were attributed to anemia. Her hemoglobin was 9.0 g%. Random blood glucose was 70 mg/dL that was attributed to poor-food intake. Limited work-up at that time revealed normocytic, normochromic anemia with normal serum iron and serum iron binding capacity. The renal functions, liver functions, and calcium profile were normal. The serum T4 was 4 µg/dL (normal: 5–12 µg/dL) and serum thyroid-stimulating hormone (TSH) was 8.0 µIU/mL. The serum sodium was 130 mEq/L and potassium was 3.9 mEq/L. The nausea prompted the physician to refer the patient to a gastroenterologist. Ultrasound of abdomen and upper gastrointestinal endoscopy were with in normal. She was told that her problems were due to mild hypothyroidism and a small dose of thyroxine 50 µg was started. However, this has worsened her symptoms and she soon stopped the thyroxine.

Past history: She attained menarche at the age of thirteen years and normal menstrual history. She was married at age of 21 years, and had four deliveries. The first three deliveries were normal, full-term vaginal deliveries and she breast-fed all the three babies for more than a year. The fourth delivery at the age of 34 years was also a full-term normal vaginal delivery, but she had profuse bleeding following child birth, and she had to undergo hysterectomy (but the ovaries were kept intact). Even though she recovered from the postpartum hemorrhage (PPH), she was unable to lactate. In the ensuing months she was placed on calcium and vitamin-D supplementation.

On further inquiry during visit with endocrinologist, patient stated that a couple of years after hysterectomy she was losing interest in sex and of late she has very poor sexual drive and libido. All along this period she had remained on calcium and vitamin-D supplements.

Physical examination: Patient was in no acute distress. She weighed 55 kg, and was 154 cm tall. Abdominal girth was 88 cm and hip circumference was measured at 86 cm. Blood pressure was 110/70 mmHg. Without orthostasis, and heart rate was 86 beats/minute. Skin was smooth and looked paler. There were no areas of hypo or hyperpigmentation. Thyroid gland was nonpalpable, and she had loss of axillary and pubic hair. Breasts were atrophic. Remainder of physical examination (neurological, cardiovascular, pulmonary, and abdomen) was unremarkable.

DIFFERENTIAL DIAGNOSIS

- Adrenal insufficiency
- Hypothyroidism
- Sheehan's syndrome (postpartum pituitary necrosis)
- Hypopituitarism from invasion or infiltration of pituitary gland (infections).

INVESTIGATIONS

- Hemoglobin: 11.2 g/dL
- White blood cell: 9,500 (poly, 40%; lymph, 49%; eos, 11%)
- Erythrocyte sedimentation rate: 40 mm/1st hour
- Fasting blood glucose: 102 mg/dL
- Blood urea nitrogen: 23.0 mg/dL
- Creatinine: 0.9 mg/dL
- Calcium: 8.8 mg/dL
- Alkaline phosphatase: 121 IU/L
- Cholesterol (total): 256 mg/dL
- Triglycerides: 213 mg/dL
- Free T4: 0.6 ng/dL (normal: 0.7–1.6 ng/dL)
- Thyroid-stimulating hormone (TSH): 0.4 µIU/mL (normal: 0.4–4.4 µIU/mL)
- Plasma cortisol: 3.4 µg/dL (normal: 7–20 µg/dL)
- Prolactin: 11.0 ng/mL (normal: 8–22 ng/mL)
- Luteinizing hormone: 0.5 mIU/mL
- Follicle-stimulating hormone: 0.9 uIU/mL
- Estradiol: <10 pg/mL.

The magnetic resonance imaging (MRI) (Brain) showed normal brain parenchyma without any mass lesions. The Pituitary fossa was reported as empty sella.

TREATMENT

This case was diagnosed as hypopituitarism, attributable to postpartum pituitary necrosis and the patient was placed on hydrocortisone (10 mg in the morning, 5 mg at noon, and 5 mg in the evening) and thyroxine 50 µg daily (early morning on an empty stomach). The patient was instructed to continue calcium and vitamin-D supplementation and it was decided not to start estrogen replacement. She was advised to monitor serum electrolytes and blood glucose periodically. She was also advised to obtain measurement of bone density by dual-energy X-ray for evaluation of bone mineral content.

DISCUSSION

Patient's history, physical findings, and investigations (laboratory and imaging studies) were suggestive of hypopituitarism. This diagnosis was initially missed owing to hysterectomy and hence absence of menses. However, failure to lactate should have been a red flag. When first physician saw this patient, he correctly identified hypothyroidism and treated as such. Over the years, the patient unfolded as a case of hypopituitarism that was quite overt by the time, the patient saw endocrinologist. Piecing together history and evolution of pituitary hypofunction, diagnosis of Sheehan's syndrome was made.

Postpartum necrosis of the pituitary (Sheehan's syndrome) or infarction of the anterior pituitary is often triggered by massive uterine hemorrhage at the time of delivery. Thanks to improved obstetric care in many parts of the world, this disorder is relatively less common now. First report of postpartum anterior pituitary necrosis dates back to 1913 (Glinsky). This was followed by report of pituitary atrophy in a woman with puerperal sepsis, who died several years later by Simmonds (1914) and it was now termed as Simmonds's disease. Later, Sheehan reported a series of case in 1937 and after his publication it came to be known as Sheehan's syndrome.

First hormonal deficiency to evolve in our case was that of prolactin as she never lactated after the episode of profuse postpartum hemorrhage (PPH). Of late the patient had developed symptoms of glucocorticoid (cortisol) deficiency manifesting as tiredness, weakness, and nausea. It is difficult to say whether she had growth hormone deficiency (GHD) since symptoms of adult GHD are very vague. For the diagnosis of hypopituitarism, clinical examination is most rewarding in children (compromise of height, weight, and pubertal status). In adults, physical examination may not be as revealing during early evolution of hypopituitarism. Of course, a careful history and examination is needed to rule out other possible etiologies of hypopituitarism. Always consider hypopituitarism in those with postpartum failure of lactation, sparse pubic and axillary hair, and involution of the breast, unexplained amenorrhea, and inability to lose weight, anemia, asthenia, and decreased libido. The pallor and gastrointestinal symptoms are probably common manifestations of hypopituitarism, which should draw the attention of treating physician. In a busy clinic, there is a tendency to attribute all symptoms to anemia. Hyponatremia, amenorrhea, and recurrent hypoglycemia are other common manifestations. Unexplained case of vomiting and upper gastrointestinal symptoms should be evaluated for cortisol deficiency. The diagnosis of hypopituitarism is based on endocrine tests ranging from measuring basal levels of all pituitary hormones, to dynamic stimulating tests of individual hormones. Mild elevations of TSH can occur in central hypothyroidism (usually high normal range). Furthermore, in a small percentage of people (10%), a modest elevation of TSH may be seen with glucocorticoid deficiency (adrenal insufficiency). It must be remembered that the relationship between TSH and T4 is logarithmic, which means that even a mild drop in circulating free T4 will cause profound elevations in TSH. An MRI of the pituitary is required for a complete diagnosis.

The etiology of hypopituitarism must be sought whenever possible. In any given case one can come to reasonable conclusion based on age of onset of symptoms and the medical history related to the development of symptoms of hypopituitarism. In this case history of PPH followed by absence of lactation provide strong clue to the possible postpartum pituitary necrosis. The pituitary gland is usually enlarged and vascular during pregnancy and with severe shock/hypotension occurring in those with PPH, there is intense spasm of the pituitary vessels resulting in severe ischemia and infarction of the gland. The infarction of the gland may be patchy and not affecting hormone production uniformly. The first clinical symptom usually is the absence of lactation as lactotrophs are most hypertrophied during pregnancy and hence most vulnerable. The extent of pituitary dysfunction following PPH is related to the size of the necrosis/infarct. There is no predetermined hierarchy for loss of hormonal function. Growth hormone deficiency has often been reported, but it may be a function of the test chosen to test rather than true hormonal deficiency. However, it should be excluded whenever possible. The severity of Sheehan's syndrome may rest on anatomical size of the sella, extent of hemorrhage, and presence of diabetes mellitus. In those evolving slowly, a possible role for antipituitary and antihypothalamic antibodies has been considered but not proven. The loss of hormone producing ability may not necessarily be permanent. Pregnancy has been reported in cases previously diagnosed as Sheehan's syndrome (but this is less common).

When diagnosis has been confirmed, missing hormone replacement should aim at improving symptoms, while avoiding overtreatment. Treatment is usually given with the target hormones rather than the deficient pituitary hormones such as glucocorticoid replacement for adrenocorticotropic hormone (ACTH) deficiency, levothyroxine for TSH deficiency, and estrogens for gonadotropin deficiency. However, in those patients with hypopituitarism desirous of fertility, treatment with gonadotropins is indicated as long as they have intact uterus and ovaries. If estrogen replacement is not considered, patient should be placed on treatments to delay or prevent bone loss (osteoporosis).

CONCLUSION

Sheehan's syndrome continues to be an important cause of hypopituitarism despite improved obstetric care in India. Anemia, hyponatremia, and hypoglycemia are often encountered. Failure to lactate, is the most common presentation, followed by thyroid dysfunction and hypoadrenalism. All women presenting with unexplained tiredness, weakness, or amenorrhea must be evaluated for hypopituitarism. Like, most endocrine diseases hypopituitarism is a great masquerader. History of PPH provides an important clue to the etiology of hypopituitarism. Properly diagnosed and adequately treated with missing hormones, a near normal, the healthy life is possible.

KEY POINTS

- In patients with history of PPH (even remote) consider hypopituitarism when symptoms like fatigue and hypoglycemia predominate
- Those with history of failure to lactate are at the highest risk for Sheehan's syndrome
- Hormonal loss may be selective and not involving all hormones necessarily
- Treatment with adequate and appropriate hormone replacement will correct all hematological and endocrine aberrations seen in patients with Sheehan's syndrome
- Full spectrum of hormonal deficiencies may take years to evolve; hence, vigilance cannot be overemphasized.

SUGGESTED READINGS

1. Kilicli F, Dokmetas SD, Acibucu F. Sheehan's syndrome. Gynecol Endocrinol. 2013;29(4):292-5.
2. Ozdogan M, Yazicioglu G, Karadogan I, et al. Sheehan's syndrome associated with pancytopenia due to marrow aplasia; full recovery with hormone replacement therapy. Int J Clin Pract. 2004;58:533-5.
3. Tessnow AH, Wilson JG. The changing face of Sheehan's syndrome. The Am J Med Sciences. 2010;340:402-6.

CHAPTER

10

Hyperparathyroidism

Sridhar R Gumpeny

CASE PRESENTATION

Case 1

A 27-year-old woman presented for evaluation of renal calculus and was observed to have a swelling in the neck during physical examination. Hypercalcemia was identified during the initial course of work-up.

Case 2

A 26-year-old woman underwent investigation for back pain. She was reported to have a mass near the region of left kidney. Initial work-up revealed hypercalcemia. She underwent further testing to establish final diagnosis and plan therapy.

DIFFERENTIAL DIAGNOSIS

Symptomatic hyperparathyroidism with hypercalcemia and renal stones is a common presentation in India, where measurement of serum calcium is not on routine investigative panel. In those Indian centers where serum calcium is routinely measured, asymptomatic hyperparathyroidism with hypercalcemia is being identified at an earlier stage of the disease.

PERTINENT INVESTIGATIONS

Case 1*:* Biochemical investigations showed elevation of serum calcium:

- Intact parathyroid hormone (iPTH): 270.6 pg/mL (normal: 11.1–79.5 pg/mL)

- Serum calcium: 13.7 mg/dL (normal: 8.0–10.2 mg/dL)
- Vitamin D (25-hydroxyvitamin D): 12 ng/mL (normal: 30–75 ng/mL)
- Serum albumin: 4.1 g/dL (normal: 4–6.0 g/dL)
- Alkaline phosphatase: 108 U/L (normal: 35–130 U/L)
- Imaging studies of the kidneys: Bilateral nephrocalcinosis.

Case 2:

- Serum calcium: 11.8 mg/dL (normal: 8.0–10.2 mg/dL)
- iPTH: 521.1 pg/mL (normal: 11.1–79.5 pg/mL)
- Alkaline phosphatase: 153 U/L (normal: 35–130 U/L)
- Plasma calcitonin: 4.78 pg/mL (normal: 5–13 pg/mL)
- 24-hour urine metanephrine: 41.77 μg (normal: <350 μg/24 hours)
- Plasma free metanephrine: 85.6 pg/dL (normal: <90 pg/dL)
- Electrolytes: Na/K: 142/3.5 mmol/L.

MANAGEMENT

Case 1 was advised to undergo parathyroid surgery in view of symptomatic hypercalcemia. A consultation with surgeon has been scheduled.

Case 2 underwent parathyroid surgery that showed multiple parathyroid adenomas in the right lower, left lower, and left upper glands; right upper gland appeared normal. Four weeks later, she underwent excision of the hypoechoic adrenal mass.

Following surgery, case 2 had normal calcium levels (below 9.5 mg/dL) until 6 months after surgery. Intact parathyroid hormone (PTH) was at the upper limit of normal (69.1 pg/mL) (normal: 15–68.3). Her serum calcium steadily rose to 10.2 mg/dL. Dual-energy X-ray absorptiometry of skeleton did not show evidence of bone loss (osteopenia or osteoporosis).

DISCUSSION

Primary hyperparathyroidism is the most common cause of hypercalcemia in clinical practice and must remain at the forefront of differential diagnosis for subjects with elevated levels of serum calcium (Boxes 10.1, 10.2). Worldwide and in developing countries still, symptomatic hyperparathyroidism and hypercalcemia presents with "moans, pains, and emotional groans." Until recently, primary hyperparathyroidism was diagnosed when symptomatic (bone involvement or renal stones), but in centers where routine screening is practiced, it is increasingly identified in the asymptomatic stages.

Box 10.1: Hyperparathyroidism

- Parathyroid adenoma (common)
  - Single gland involvement (common), multiple adenomas
- Parathyroid hyperplasia
- As part of MEN syndromes/familial forms
- Carcinoma (rare)

Box 10.2: Causes of hypercalcemia

- Endocrine causes
  - Hyperparathyroidism (primary, tertiary)
  - Adrenal insufficiency
  - Thyrotoxicosis
  - Acromegaly
- Neoplastic causes (lymphoma, T-cell leukemia]
- Other causes
  - Granulomatous disorders (sarcoidosis, histoplasmosis, etc.)
  - Paget's disease
  - Immobilization
  - Lithium intake
  - Aquired immunodeficiency syndrome

ETIOLOGY AND PRESENTATION

Epidemiology

In the United States, an estimated 1,00,000 new patients are diagnosed with primary hyperparathyroidism each year. This reflects earlier diagnosis and tilting balance toward asymptomatic hyperparathyroidism rather than classic symptomatic state. This not different from what is increasingly being reported from major metropolitan centers worldwide.

Inappropriately normal or increased parathormone [(parathyroid hormone) (iPTH)] secretion occurs most commonly from a single-gland adenoma in nearly 4–5th of cases, [four-gland hyperplasia (10–15%), and rarely from a carcinoma]. Parathyroid adenomas occur more often in the lower pole; they range in size from 1–3 cm and weigh 0.3 g to 4–5 g. Ectopic adenomas are uncommon may be found embedded with the thymus. Hyperparathyroidism is a disease of increased age, with a reported prevalence of 1% in adults and 2% in those over the age of 55. Peak prevalence occurs in the seventh decade, more often in women, but there is equal sex distribution below the age of 45. Epidemiological studies in India have been plagued by very high background vitamin D deficiency, lack of patient registries, and paucity of facilities for thorough and reliable measurement of vitamin D and PTH levels. These difficulties, largely technical, are being addressed in emerging centers of excellence located mostly in larger cities.

Risk Factors

There are few recognized risk factors for hyperparathyroidism, except for irradiation of head and neck during childhood as in treatment for acne, or in survivors of atomic bomb, as well as use of lithium over long time. It may be seen as part of multiple endocrine neoplasia syndromes (types 1 and 2A; mostly former).

Indian Scenario

In a 2011 systematic review of publications on primary hyperparathyroidism from India, 858 individuals were reported between the years 1980 and 2010. Most were from Institutions with special research focus on bone and metabolism disorders. Over time, the number of publications tended to increase, although far fewer than those from developed countries, suggesting that awareness about the condition was increasing. There was female preponderance (1.7:1) of younger age (<70% were below the age of 40 years), and the symptoms occurred for a mean of nearly seven years (84 months). Most cases are sporadic. Familial cases occur as part of multiple endocrine neoplasia syndromes.

These earlier studies identified mostly symptomatic cases at advanced stage that often came to the attention of orthopedic surgeons and urologists first, while being worked up for fractures and renal stones. In decreasing order the involvement following presentations were recorded: bone disease, proximal muscle weakness, brown tumors, fractures, renal disease, psychiatric symptoms, pancreatitis, and asymptomatic. Lately in contrast, asymptomatic disease accounted for >80% of cases, with only 15% with renal disease, 5% with bone disease, and 3% with brown tumors. Where vitamin D levels were measured, they were low in Indian patients (10.21 + 5.82 ng/mL). With increasing use of screening in asymptomatic individuals, earlier and therefore, milder forms of hyperparathyroidism are being identified. In a recent report from a paying hospital, the proportion of subjects with fractures, brown tumors, and psychiatric manifestations was lower. Among 52 patients reported from Postgraduate Institute of Medical Education and Research (PGIMER), Chandigarh, India, hypercalcemia (86.5%) and hypophosphatemia (65.4%) were prominent. Those with nephrocalcinosis only had lower levels of PTH than those with bone disease. "Hungry bone disease" was found in a little over half.

What about the "*Indian variant*"? It is mostly a non-issue since Indians settled abroad for generations do not have a distinctly different course or biochemical presentation. Shortage of milk and mass malnutrition in decades preceding increase in domestic milk production and consumption would have negatively impacted regulation of calcium and iPTH in the Indian subcontinent.

Evidence is available for a possible modulation by vitamin D levels. A study showed that in countries where milk was fortified with vitamin D, there was a decline of parathyroid tumor weight as well as the prevalence of osteitis fibrosa. In contrast countries without fortification showed little change in both. It is possible that the high rates of vitamin D deficiency in India could alter the clinical expression as well as the tumor growth of parathyroid glands. This is reflected by studies from India published in 2001, where the mean iPTH and total alkaline phosphatase levels were elevated by nearly 15 times normal in subjects who presented with severe symptomatic disease involving the skeleton, muscle, and kidneys in young subjects.

Clinical Manifestations

Depending on the methods employed for identification, primary hyperparathyroidism can present from asymptomatic hypercalcemia to symptomatic hypercalcemia with involvement of bones, kidneys, and muscles (Box 10.3).

Symptoms may be nonspecific, such as complaints of weakness, fatigue, anxiety, or cognitive impairment. The prevalence of fractures increases,

Box 10.3: Presenting features of hyperparathyroidism

- Asymptomatic
- Clinical features related to:
  - Skeletal system
    - Bone pain, arthralgia, particularly of legs
    - Low bone density
    - Pathological fractures
  - Neuromuscular
    - Muscle cramps
    - Paresthesias
  - Cardiovascular
    - Hypertension
    - Electrocardiogram alterations: Prolonged P–R interval; short Q–T interval
  - Gastrointestinal
    - Appetite loss
    - Abdominal pain
    - Constipation

and can be predicted by lower bone mineral density (BMD), particularly in cortical bones such as distal radius. Hypertension and related cardiac risk factors are also present.

Elevated PTH without Hypercalcemia

Particularly among those investigated for low BMD, there may be elevated levels of PTH without hypercalcemia. This "normocalcemic primary hyperparathyroidism" must be diagnosed only after ruling other causes of hyperparathyroidism, particularly secondary causes.

Another condition to be differentiated where hypercalcemia and modest elevation of PTH occurs is "familial benign hypocalciuric hypercalcemia." This is often identified only after failed parathyroidectomy for presumed primary hyperparathyroidism. It is an autosomal dominant condition due to a functional mutation (loss of function) of *CaSR* gene (that encodes calcium sensing receptor) located on chromosome 3. A family history of hypercalcemia and failed neck surgery should raise the suspicion of this condition. The 24-hour urinary calcium and creatinine levels should be measured. A calcium/creatinine clearance ratio below 0.01 helps establish diagnosis.

Normoparathyroid Hypercalcemia

Recently a Danish group reported a new subgroup of patients who has baseline high calcium levels with normal iPTH. These patients later progress to primary hyperparathyroidism. Unlike their normocalcemic hyperparathyroid counterparts, patients do not have altered baseline vitamin D metabolism. Interestingly parathyroid hyperplasia is more common histopathological finding in this group, whereas parathyroid adenoma is more common in patients with normocalcemic hyperparathyroidism.

NATURAL COURSE

The natural history depends on the severity of hyperparathyroidism. If it is severe and the patient has symptoms, absence of surgical intervention leads to worsening of disease, particularly renal stones. On the other hand if the disease is mild (serum calcium <1 mg/dL above the normal range), follow-up studies up to 8 years showed that biochemical parameters could be stationary. However, nearly a third have worsening of hypercalcemia and lowering of bone density. Similarly the risk of cardiovascular mortality is also increased that persists beyond successful parathyroidectomy.

Therefore, one must evaluate each person independently and take a decision on the line of management. Recent evidence suggests level of parathormone at baseline (and not the level of calcium) could better predict the long-term outcome of untreated primary hyperparathyroidism.

Biochemical/Laboratory Investigations

Elevated serum calcium level is often the first evidence to suspect primary hyperparathyroidism (Box 10.4). Assessment of corrected or ionized calcium is necessary because total serum calcium is a combination of free and albumin-bound calcium. Alterations in the level of serum albumin can therefore give rise to spuriously low or high values of total serum calcium which may not be reflective of free or active form of calcium. Furthermore ionized calcium is pH sensitive and this must be taken into account when interpreting results.

Corrected total calcium is derived as follows: It is equal to (measured total calcium expressed in mg/dL) + 0.8 × (4 - patient's serum albumin concentration expressed in g/dL). In special cases, serum-ionized calcium is measured as in hyperalbuminemia, thrombocytosis, or myeloma.

The next diagnostic step consists of measuring serum PTH level. A combination of elevated serum calcium along with either elevated or "inappropriately normal" value of iPTH is indicative of primary hyperparathyroidism. Both second and third-generation PTH assays may be used. Similar findings may also be seen in other conditions such as tertiary hyperparathyroidism found in end-stage renal disease and in familial hypocalciuric hypercalcemia. The latter can be suspected on the basis of family history. If the level of serum PTH is low, it generally excludes the possibility of primary hyperparathyroidism; one must consider rarer causes such as cancer-associated hypercalcemia, mediated by PTH-related protein (PTH-rp). High iPTH may be seen with ectopic tumoral production of PTH. Vitamin D deficiency should be identified and treated.

Box 10.4: Diagnosis of hyperparathyroidism

- Symptomatic or routine biochemical screening of serum calcium
  - Confirm hypercalcemia
  - Rule out other causes or factitious hypercalcemia
- Parathyroid hormone (elevated)
- Imaging of parathyroid gland (surgical localization)
  - Ultrasound (preoperative, intraoperative)
  - Radionuclide scan
  - Computed tomography

Measurement of serum phosphorus should be routinely obtained. It is often low or normal as a consequence of PTH phosphaturia. Additionally, complete blood count and a basic metabolic panel (BMP) should be obtained as well. Law-grade anemia is not uncommon particularly with longer duration of hyperparathyroid stage. Since PTH leads to renal loss of bicarbonate, low normal serum bicarbonate level, and higher corresponding serum chloride level (>102 mmol/L) is often encountered. Where facilities are available both 25 hydroxy vitamin D (25 OHD) and 1:25 dihydroxy vitamin (1:25 OH_2D) levels must be measured. Levels of 1:25 OH_2D are elevated because of activation of 1α-hydroxylase activity in states of low phosphate and high PTH levels.

Thus, a common biochemical pattern would be seen in cases of primary hyperparathyroidism:

- Hypercalcemia
- Hypophosphatemia
- Elevated iPTH
- Increased 1:25 dihydroxy vitamin D level
- Elevated serum chloride (>102 mmol/L)
- Low normal plasma bicarbonate
- Chloride to phosphorus ratio >35.

Familial Forms

Familial forms of primary hyperparathyroidism occur in <5%, but must be considered especially when the diagnosis is made before the age of 30 years, neuroendocrine tumors, skin lesions indicative of multiple endocrine neoplasia (MEN) syndrome (types 1 and 2A). Serum calcium must be measured in all first-degree relatives. Other familial syndromes of hyperparathyroidism include:

- Hyperparathyroidism jaw tumor syndrome
- Familial hypocalciuric hypercalcemia
- Neonatal severe primary hyperparathyroidism
- Familial isolated hyperparathyroidism.

Renal Function and Further Specialized Tests

Both renal function and levels of (25 OHD) must be assessed to rule out renal insufficiency and vitamin D deficiency, which is common in Indian population. Many centers will routinely measure 1:25 OH_2D levels as well. A BMP often provides information on electrolyte status that can help in diagnosis. Serum phosphorus measurement must be obtained whenever possible.

Where possible and necessary and paid for, sequencing of calcium-sensing receptor gene may be considered in familial hypocalciuric hypercalcemia.

Imaging Studies

Once hyperparathyroidism has been confirmed to be the cause of hypercalcemia, the source of elevated PTH must be sought. Imaging of the neck is often not indicated for localization before surgery. However, sestamibi (MIBI) scanning and ultrasound may be employed, with the former having the advantage of locating ectopic parathyroid glands. A recent publication concluded that localization of parathyroid gland is indicated where surgery is planned on the parathyroid glands. One must consider related issues such as availability of facilities and expertise, the cost involved and accuracy.
Imaging of kidneys and bones:

- In the presence of renal stones, imaging would have preceded the identification of primary hyperparathyroidism. A recent clinical review concluded that all subjects with primary hyperparathyroidism should undergo imaging study for renal calcification; if stones are present, parathyroidectomy is advised. In those who develop renal stones after parathyroidectomy, the evaluation and treatment is similar to other patients with renal stones
- The same holds true for subjects presenting with bone involvement. Even in those who are asymptomatic, BMD measurement is advised at the lumbar spine, hip, and forearm because reduced cortical bone density is expected in primary hyperparathyroidism.

TREATMENT OPTIONS

Asymptomatic Primary Hyperparathyroidism

An international workshop on management of asymptomatic primary hyperparathyroidism held in 2008 provided guidelines. It should be emphasized that individuals with biochemically confirmed primary hyperparathyroidism with specific symptoms or signs need surgery. Medical monitoring without surgery is an option for a subgroup with asymptomatic primary hyperparathyroidism.

Suggested indications for parathyroid surgery:

- Serum calcium: >1 mg/dL above upper limit of normal
- Calculated creatinine clearance: <60 mL/min

- BMD: T score < –2.5 at lumber spine, or total hip or femoral neck or distal one third site of radius, and/or previous fracture
- Age: <50 years.

Unlike earlier recommendations, 24-hour urinary calcium estimation is not routinely indicated.

If the patient is an appropriate candidate for follow-up, without the need for immediate surgery, the following guidelines apply:

1. Annual measurement of serum calcium
2. Annual measurement of serum creatinine
3. Annual or biannual measurement of bone density, at three sites.

Indication for parathyroidectomy even in asymptomatic hyperparathyroidism gained strength because over time, bone density appeared to get worse, and because surgical removal of parathyroid glands would reduce the remaining lifetime fracture risk. This needs confirmation by randomized clinical trials.

In general, majority of patients may eventually need surgery, particularly among those with low or falling bone density. Outcome of cardiovascular events and of cognitive function is not established. Because of falling bone density over time, age below 50 years has been considered an indication for surgery.

Surgical Treatment

The goal of surgery is to remove all abnormal parathyroid tissue to cure the disease. All symptomatic subjects should be recommended to undergo parathyroidectomy. The most important outcome predictor has been described as choosing the right surgeon, one with experience and skill in exploring the anatomical regions, identifying gland abnormalities, and carefully removing the abnormal gland tissue. The standard treatment is "full-neck exploration with identification of all glands." A clean and successful first surgery is most desirable. Reoperation following poorly done primary surgery is always a compromise even in the best of hands. The surgeon's skill and decision-making are important, rather than the surgical procedure itself. Experienced surgeons can achieve a cure rate >95%. Intraoperative PTH monitoring and ultrasound for locating parathyroid glands are also available. Recurrence is rare in sporadic hyperparathyroidism, in contrast to familial cases.

Indian surgeons approached the glands by bilateral or unilateral neck exploration, while some did focused parathyroidectomy; the last in patients with concordant ultrasound and MIBI findings. Recurrence occurred in none to about 4% and persistent hyperparathyroidism in none to about 2.5; weight of parathyroid tumor in India ranges from 1 to 100 g.

Postoperative Course and Long-Term Prognosis

In India, postoperative hungry bone syndrome was reported in a quarter to nearly three fourths of subjects who underwent surgery. They have early symptomatic hypocalcemia or biochemical hypocalcemia following parathyroidectomy. The maximum fall occurred between 12 and 33 hours after surgery. Intravenous calcium infusion may be required for 3–8 days. In addition oral carbonate in a dose of 2 g/day and calcitriol (1 μg/day) may be required. Reported mortality rates from India were up to 7%, with half due to end-stage renal disease and to metastatic disease. It was high in those having kidney stone disease.

One of the earlier reports of parathyroidectomy from India described that following surgery, osteitis fibrosa cystica resolves early and to a marked degree. Recovery at cancellous bone at the spine is prompt as seen by bone density studies; cortical bone at forearm does not recover as promptly. If the disease is severe, defects of contour may persist, which require corrective osteotomies.

Persistent or Recurrent Primary Hyperparathyroidism

Uncommon, though it is in experienced hands, persistent, or recurrent primary hyperparathyroidism is a clinical challenge. *Persistent* primary hyperparathyroidism is often due to inadequate removal of the pathological tissue. It is often due to difficulty in locating and excising a parathyroid adenoma. A repeat surgical exploration is often necessary. In contrast, *recurrent* primary hyperparathyroidism is far less common: here a subject has had successful initial surgery as defined by normal serum PTH and calcium levels for at least 6 months following surgery and then develops recurrence of the disease. Both persistent and recurrent primary hyperparathyroidism are more often seen in MEN syndromes.

A careful re-evaluation is necessary in these conditions. Efforts must be made to exclude drug induced alterations of calcium levels (e.g. lithium and thiazides), other causes of elevated PTH levels such as secondary causes following renal insufficiency, renal calcium loss, vitamin D deficiency, and gastrointestinal abnormalities. A careful 24-hour measurement of calcium excretion is necessary to identify familial benign hypocalciuric hypercalcemia.

In addition, a careful family history can help in establishing diagnosis. Families with familial benign hypocalciuric hypercalcemia are generally asymptomatic, whereas those with multiple endocrine neoplasia type 1 syndrome (MEN1) have primary hyperparathyroidism before the age of 30 and have recurrent disease. The course of MEN2 is dominated mostly by medullary carcinoma of thyroid and pheochromocytoma rather than hyperparathyroidism. Formal genetic testing for the MEN syndromes may be indicated where available.

A rule of thumb for surgery is that threshold for surgery must be higher because of the difficulty in reoperation. However, it must not be withheld when significant symptoms and signs are found. Imaging modalities are of value in such situations. A suggested sequence consists of neck ultrasound, followed sestamibi with single-photon emission computed tomography (CT), a 4D CT scan, and going on to ultrasound aspiration of suspected neck lesion or venous localization by a skilled radiographic specialist. Surgery requires "both judgment and technique" on the part of surgeon.

Medical Management of Primary Hyperparathyroidism

In those subjects who are not fit or who are unwilling to undergo surgery, yet in whom serum calcium levels must be lowered, a trial of drugs may be attempted. Although estrogen replacement treatment is on the wane, conjugated estrogen (0.625 mg) and medroxyprogesterone (5 mg) for two years increased BMD. Similarly alendronate (20 mg) for 2 years increased BMD. Where the issue is not of low BMD, but elevated serum calcium levels *cinacalcet* is approved for use. It is an expensive treatment.

KEY POINTS

- Primary hyperparathyroidism is still being identified in late in its clinical course (renal stones, bone fractures, brown tumors, non-specific symptoms) where routine screening of serum calcium is not done
- Elevated serum calcium (total and ionized) along with elevated or inappropriately normal PTH levels and low serum phosphorus confirms the diagnosis
- All symptomatic subjects should be offered surgical removal of parathyroid adenoma (which is the commonest cause of primary hyperparathyroidism)
- Choice of an experienced surgeon is important
- Concomitant vitamin D deficiency should be corrected to prevent postoperative hungry bone syndrome
- Following successful surgery, recurrence is unusual; if it occurs, familial forms of MEN syndromes should be considered.

SUGGESTED READINGS

1. Augustine MM, Bravo PE, Zeiger MA. Surgical treatment of primary hyperparathyroidism. Endocrine Pract 2011 (Suppl 1); 17:75-82.
2. Bilezikian JP, Khan AA, Potts JT, et al. Guidelines for the management of asymptomatic primary hyperparathyroidism: summary statement—3rd international workshop. J Clin Endocrinol Metab. 2009;94:335-9.
3. Kunstman JW, Kirsch JD, Mahajan A, et al. Parathyroid localization and implications for clinical management. J Clin Endocrinol Metab. 2013;98:902-12.
4. Marocci C, Cetani F. Primary hyperparathyroidism. N Engl J Med. 2011;365:2389-97.
5. Mishra SK, Agarwal G, Kar DJ, et al. Unique clinical characteristics of primary hyperparathyroidism in India. Br J Surg. 2001;88:708-14.
6. Rejnmark L, Vestergaard P, Mosekilde L. Nephrolithiasis and renal calcifications in primary hyperparathyroidism. J Clin Endocrinol Metab. 2011;96:2377-85.
7. Udelsman R. Approach to the patient with persistent or recurrent primary hyperparathyroidism. J Clin Endocinol Metab. 2011;96:2950.
8. Yu N, Leese GP, Donnan PT. What predicts adverse outcomes in untreated primary hyperparathyroidism? The Parathyroid Epidemiology and Audit Research Study (PEARS). Clin Endocrinol. 2013;79:27-34.

CHAPTER

11

Diabetic Ketoacidosis with Cerebral Edema

Siddhnath Sudhanshu, Vijayalakshmi Bhatia, Eesh Bhatia

CASE PRESENTATION

An 11-year-old boy was brought to the emergency room with rapid breathing of 8 hour duration. He had been symptomatic for the last 10 days in the form of polyuria, polydipsia, tiredness, and weight loss. Since the previous 24 hours, he was complaining of abdominal pain and had two episodes of vomiting. Parents did not give any history of fever, cough, altered sensorium, or any similar episode in the past. The child was passing urine at regular intervals. He was previously not known to have diabetes mellitus.

CLINICAL AND LABORATORY DATA

At the time of presentation, he was severely dehydrated. His pulses were palpable with pulse rate 120 beats/minute. His blood pressure was 100/70 mmHg. His respiration was deep and rapid with a respiratory rate of 44 breaths/minute. The child was afebrile and his chest was bilaterally clear to auscultation. He had normal sensorium with equally and normally reacting pupils. The rest of his general physical and systemic examination was normal.

On further evaluation and investigations, the patient had high blood glucose (BG >500 mg/dL) with severe high anion gap metabolic acidosis (pH: 7.04; HCO_3^-: 5.3 mEq/L). Blood ketones by ketone strip were 2.4 mmol/L. Electrocardiogram (ECG) did not show any U wave or tall T waves. Potassium level in the venous blood gas (VBG) was 3.22 mEq/L.

DIFFERENTIAL DIAGNOSIS: POLYURIA, POLYDIPSIA, DEHYDRATION, AND WEIGHT LOSS

- Diabetes mellitus
- Diabetes insipidus
- Severe gastrointestinal fluid loss of any etiology.

The combination of polyuria, polydipsia, and hyperglycemia is a strong indicator of diabetes mellitus (although mild hyperglycemia may be seen in any acute nondiabetic sickness—stress hyperglycemia).

When combined with moderate-to-strong metabolic acidosis and ketonemia, diabetic ketoacidosis (DKA) must be diagnosed unless proven otherwise. It is a medical emergency and must be attended to immediately. Diagnosis can be further substantiated by measurement of glycated hemoglobin. A nonemergent measurement glutamic acid decarboxylase (GAD-65) antibody would help confirm diagnosis of type-1 diabetes.

MANAGEMENT

The patient was given 400 mL of normal saline as a bolus, intravenously over 1 hour by the emergency room personnel between the time an endocrinologist saw him. The patient was diagnosed to have severe DKA with severe dehydration and was admitted. He was started on intravenous fluid infusion of normal saline with added potassium (40 mEq/L). His weight was 45 kg at the time of admission. The rate of fluid administration was calculated as follows: fluid deficit was calculated as 80 mL/kg to be given evenly over the next 48 hours along with the maintenance fluid for the duration; from this was subtracted the bolus fluid volume of 400 mL given in the emergency room. After 1 hour of starting the intravenous fluid infusion, repeat VBG report showed pH to be 7.1, bicarbonate 5.2, and potassium 3.54 mEq/L. Repeat ECG did not show any abnormality. Insulin infusion was then started at the rate of 0.1 unit/kg/h.

Samples for serum electrolytes, creatinine, liver function tests, blood culture, hemoglobin, and total leukocyte count were sent. He was catheterized and was seen to be passing urine adequately.

Investigation reports revealed serum creatinine to be 1.2 mg/dL, hemoglobin 13.4 g/dL, TLC 10,900/mm^3; serum sodium 142 mEq/L, serum potassium 3.6 mEq/L, and liver function tests to be within normal limits. Chest X-ray showed clear lung fields.

The dehydration, acidosis, and blood glucose improved over the next few hours; however, after 8 hours the child appeared drowsy and lethargic. He was arousable only by light pain. His blood pressure (BP) had risen to

132/84 mmHg and his heart rate (HR) had slowed down to 80/minute. Repeat VBG report revealed pH 7.2, bicarbonate 8.1 mEq/L, sodium 146 mEq/L, and potassium 3.5 mEq/L. A diagnosis of cerebral edema was made due to worsened sensorium and relative slowing of HR and rise in blood pressure. A single infusion of Mannitol (0.5 g/kg) was given over 20 minutes. The sensorium improved dramatically within an hour of mannitol infusion. A repeat infusion was not required.

He was switched to 0.45% saline 5% dextrose when blood glucose touched 250 mg%. After 22 hours, he was hungry and fully alert. Bowel sounds were normal. He was allowed to eat meals, the insulin infusion being increased to cover meal related glucose excursions. The patient recovered from metabolic acidosis after a total of 36 hours, and only then he was put on subcutaneous basal bolus insulin injection regimen with glargine and regular insulin. He was found to have hypophosphatemia that got corrected spontaneously after shifting to oral feeds. He required oral potassium chloride for 4 days.

Diabetes education was given to the patient and the parents. He is in regular follow-up and doing well in school. He is performing self-monitoring of blood glucose and making insulin dose adjustment appropriately.

DISCUSSION

Diabetic ketoacidosis may be the initial presentation in about one third of newly diagnosed patients with diabetes mellitus. Severity is inversely related to age at the time of presentation, thus making younger children most vulnerable. Although DKA is most often seen in patients with type-1 diabetes, increasingly it is also being recognized in children with type-2 diabetes mellitus. This may be a consequence of acute, rapid metabolic decompensation, akin to that seen in adults (Flatbush Diabetes) in the setting of insulin resistance. Diabetic ketoacidosis is a potentially life-threatening complication of diabetes mellitus.

Diagnostic Criteria

- Hyperglycemia (blood glucose >200 mg/dL)
- Venous pH <7.3 or bicarbonate <15 mmol/L
- Presence of ketones in blood and urine.

Severity of Diabetic Ketoacidosis

- Mild: Venous pH < 7.3, bicarbonate <15 mmol/L
- Moderate: Venous pH < 7.2, bicarbonate <10 mmol/L
- Severe: Venous pH < 7.1, bicarbonate <5 mmol/L.

The basic pathophysiology of DKA in children is same as in adults, but the child differs from the adult in a number of characteristics including rapid deterioration, and risk of cerebral edema in diabetic ketoacidosis (CEDKA). Fundamentally, DKA reflects a state of cellular starvation amidst surfeit of fuel unable to satisfy energy requirements of cell because of lack of insulin and/or insulin resistance. In order to meet metabolic needs, body attempts to utilize adipose tissue as the main source of energy. However, lack of insulin leads to overproduction of acetyl-CoA (under normal circumstances acetyl-CoA pairs with oxaloacetate to enter tricarboxylic cycle. In states of decreased oxaloacetate such as the DKA, acetyl-CoA metabolism will be shifted toward ketone body production). The acetoacetate generated from acetyl-CoA is converted directly to β-hydroxy butyric acid (BHA) and acetone both of which are ketone bodies. In DKA with reduced mitochondrial redox state [nicotinamide adenine dinucleotide ($NADH/NAD^+$ ratio)], the BHA and acetoacetate ratio is tilted in favor of BHA overproduction (normal ratio 1:1, ratio during DKA 10:1 or higher). Ketone bodies being strong acids dissociate freely leading to overproduction of hydrogen ions. This overproduction of hydrogen ions quickly overwhelms the buffering capacity of body leading to metabolic acidosis. Prime mover for DKA is the excess of glucagon rather than lack of insulin. This is conclusively established by resolution of DKA with continuous somatostatin infusion. However, this should be treated as proof of concept rather than assuming insulin being totally dispensable when treating DKA. Insulin treatment continues to remain standard of care for now.

Management of DKA involves fluid resuscitation to rehydrate and improve tissue perfusion (importantly renal perfusion); correction of ketoacidosis and hyperglycemia by inhibiting ketogenesis and enhancing tissue glucose uptake by administration of insulin; resolution of electrolyte imbalance; and avoidance of complications such as hypoglycemia. A vital fact to keep in mind while managing DKA is that cerebral and other autoregulatory mechanisms may not be as well developed in younger children. This may predispose to severe therapy related complications in children with severe DKA.

Cerebral Edema

Cerebral edema in DKA is associated with significant mortality and morbidity. Population based clinical studies have shown the risk of developing cerebral edema in 0.5–1% of pediatric DKA episodes. It has a high mortality rate 21–24% and 15–26% of the survivors are left with permanent neurological sequelae. The incidence of cerebral edema in newly diagnosed cases has been found to be higher (12/1,000 DKA episodes) than in established cases (4/1,000 DKA cases) of insulin-dependent diabetes. Clinically significant cerebral edema usually develops 4–12 hours after treatment has started, but may occur even before treatment occasionally.

Pathophysiology

The exact mechanism is still not completely understood but can be attributed to several factors:

- Metabolic acidosis and ketosis may cause cytotoxic cerebral edema by inducing proinflammatory cytokines even before initiation of the treatment
- Increased blood-brain barrier permeability due to generation of various inflammatory mediators and disruption of cell membrane ion transport channels, when coupled with increased cerebral blood flow due to immature cerebral autoregulation and superimposed aggressive fluid therapy, results in cerebral edema
- Another contributing factor is intracellular osmoles generated by brain cells to counter dehydration. When plasma osmolarity falls during intensive fluid therapy and rapid fall in blood glucose due to simultaneous insulin therapy, these osmoles attract fluid and result in cerebral edema.

It is now believed that the original insult might be more vasogenic (blood-brain barrier) and that cytotoxic injury is secondary.

Warning Signs of Cerebral Edema

- Headache
- Slowing of HR, rising blood pressure
- Altered sensorium
- Fall in oxygen saturation.

Diagnostic Criteria

- Abnormal motor or verbal response to pain
- Cranial nerve palsy (especially III, IV, and VI)
- Decortication or decerebration
- Abnormal respiratory pattern like Cheyne-Stoke respiration, apneusis, or grunting.

Major Criteria

- Fluctuating level of consciousness
- Sustained HR deceleration. (Decrease >20 bpm), not attributable to improved intravascular volume or sleep state
- Age-inappropriate incontinence.

Minor Criteria

- Headache, vomiting
- Lethargy, not easily arousable
- Diastolic blood pressure >90 mmHg
- Age <5 years.

One diagnostic criterion, two major criteria, or one major and two minor criteria have a sensitivity of 92% and a false positive rate of only 4%.

A height, weight, and gender appropriate chart with the reference ranges for blood pressure should be available at the bedside. Complaints of headache should be taken seriously. A combination of hypertension, bradycardia, and irregular respiration (*Cushing triad*) reflects increased intracranial pressure.

It should be noted that cerebral edema is exclusive to pediatric patients. Cerebral lesions in fatal DKA were reported almost a century ago (Dillon et al. 1936). Young age, new-onset diabetes, severe hypocapnia (PCO_2 <20 mmHg); severe metabolic acidosis, initial fluid resuscitation of >50 mL/kg in first 4 hours, higher blood urea nitrogen at presentation, bicarbonate administration, administration of insulin in first hour of fluid resuscitation, and slower increase in measured sodium concentration during treatment of DKA have all been cited as potential risk factors.

Prevention and Therapy of Cerebral Edema

- Do not give saline bolus unless the child is hypotensive
- Administer the fluid deficit over next 48 hours along with the maintenance fluid. Deduct the amount of fluid if any, given prior to the current treatment, from the total calculated fluid, including intravenous fluids given at another health care facility
- Start insulin after 1 hour of initiation of fluid therapy to prevent sudden fall in blood glucose and the plasma osmolality. Bolus insulin at start of therapy is not recommended in children
- Do not wait for computed tomography scan to confirm cerebral edema, rely on the clinical diagnostic factors
- For treatment, give mannitol 0.5–1 g/kg IV over 20 minutes and repeat if there is no initial response in 30 minutes to 2 hours
- One should always check whether the patient is passing urine or not, before starting the mannitol infusion, else, mannitol infusion in an oliguric patient may worsen the renal failure
- In a patient with hyponatremia or coagulopathy, hypertonic saline can be used instead of mannitol.

KEY POINTS

- Cerebral edema is a therapy related complication of DKA and is associated with high mortality and morbidity
- Intravenous bolus fluid administration is not recommended unless the patient is hypotensive or in shock. In the context of the above presented case, the child was given normal saline bolus in the emergency room, which should not have been given as the patient was normotensive. This could be a risk factor for predisposing the child for development of cerebral edema
- One should have a high index of suspicion for cerebral edema in a patient with DKA if there is a change in sensorium. A careful monitoring of vitals is necessary to pick up the early signs of rising intracranial tension in the form of slowing down of heart rate and rising blood pressure
- If the patient has clinical signs of cerebral edema, he/she should be treated with mannitol infusion without delay. It is not always necessary to have central nervous system imaging for confirmation of the cerebral edema, as it may delay treatment and increase the risk of cerebral edema related mortality and morbidity
- Use of bicarbonate in severe DKA is not recommended routinely. In the presented case, bicarbonate therapy was not given even in the presence of severe acidosis. Severe acidosis in a patient with DKA is found to be reversible with insulin infusion and fluid therapy as insulin prevents further ketones production and fluid therapy improves tissue perfusion and renal excretion of organic acids. Inadvertent use of bicarbonate may lead to rapid correction of acidosis, thereby increasing the risk of severe hypokalemia. Further, there is a risk of increasing cerebral acidosis. However, cautious use of bicarbonates may benefit in selected conditions. These include patients with severe hyperkalemia and patients with severe metabolic acidosis with pH < 6.9 and hypotension after 1 hour of rehydration. When indicated, bicarbonate is used cautiously in a dose of 1–2 mmol/kg, given as slow infusion over 60 minutes. It can be added to half normal saline or water for injection to make up a solution of 150 mEq/L sodium
- Use of phosphate in the presence of hypophosphatemia is another controversial issue. ISPAD guidelines recommend use of phosphate only in the setting of severe hypophosphatemia with unexplained muscular weakness as many prospective studies have not shown clinical benefit from phosphate replacement. Phosphate administration is associated with risk of development of severe hypocalcemia, so close monitoring of serum calcium level must be done while on phosphate replacement therapy in a patient with DKA. The above presented patient had initially been found to be having hypophosphatemia but he did not have any muscular weakness. Therefore, he was not started on phosphate replacement.

SUGGESTED READINGS

1. Dalton RR, Hoffman WH, Passmore GG, et al. Plasma C-reactive protein levels in severe diabetic ketoacidosis. Ann Clin Lab Sci. 2003;33(4):435-42.
2. Edge JA, Hawkins MM, Winter DL, et al. The risk and outcome of cerebral oedema developing during diabetic ketoacidosis. Arch Dis Child. 2001;85(1):16-22.
3. Hoon EJ, Carlotti AP, Costa LA, et al. Preventing a drop in effective plasma osmolality to minimize the likelihood of cerebral edema during treatment of children with diabetic ketoacidosis. J Pediatr. 2007; 150(5):467-73.
4. ISPAD Clinical Practice Consensus Guidelines (2014) Compendium. Pediatr Diabetes. 2014;15 (suppl 20): 154-79.
5. Olivieri L, Chasm R. Diabetic Ketoacidosis in the Pediatric emergency Department. Emerg Med Clin N Am. 2013;31:755-73.
6. Roberts JS, Vavilala MS, Schenkman KA, et al. Cerebral hyperaemia and impaired cerebral autoregulation associated with diabetic ketoacidosis in critically ill children. Crit Care Med. 2006;34(8):2217-23.
7. Wolfsdorf J, Glaser N, Sperling MA. American Diabetes Association: Diabetic ketoacidosis in infants, children, and adolescents: a consensus statement from the American Diabetes Association. Diabetes Care. 2006; 29(5):1150-9.

CHAPTER

12

Polycystic Ovarian Syndrome

Mir Iftikhar Bashir, Abdul H Zargar

CASE PRESENTATION

A 19-year-old woman presented for evaluation of oligomenorrhea and hirsutism. She is product of consanguineous marriage. Patient attained menarche at age 13 years. Menstrual cycles were irregular (cycle length ranging from 35 to 90 days) from the onset. She noticed mild facial growth at about the time of menarche, first over the upper lip and chin. At age 15 years, the patient was evaluated by a gynecologist for persistent oligomenorrhea and was prescribed an oral contraceptive pill (OCP). She had regular withdrawal bleeds and hirsutism improved after OCP use. She stopped treatment on her own 2 years later assuming that she had been cured of disease.

At present she continues to have oligomenorrhea and has noticed slow progression of hair growth over face, chest, and abdomen. She does not give history of acne, alopecia, or galactorrhea. Patient also denies intake of any other medications. Her mother has type-2 diabetes, and does not give history of oligomenorrhea/hirsutism. However, patient's younger sister has similar complaints since menarche 1 year back. Patient and her mother are concerned about the oligomenorrhea and hirsutism as well as future effects on fertility.

PHYSICAL EXAMINATION

Height 165 cm; weight 82 kg [body mass index (BMI) 30.12 kg/m^2]; waist circumference (WC) 98 cm. Heart rate 86 beats/minute; blood pressure: 140/82 mmHg.

Systemic physical examination is unremarkable otherwise (no evidence of acanthosis nigricans, acne or purplish abdominal striae). Ferriman-Gallwey hirsutism score is 14 (normal <8).

LABORATORY INVESTIGATIONS

- Thyroid-stimulating hormone: 2.43 mIU/L
- FT4: 1.1 ng/dL
- Serum prolactin: 14.5 ng/mL
- Luteinizing hormone (LH): 13.4 mIU/L
- Follicle-stimulating hormone (FSH): 4.8 mIU/L
- Dehydroepiandrosterone sulfate (DHEAS): 347 μg/dL
- Total testosterone: 78 ng/dL
- Basal serum 17(OH) progesterone level: 1.5 ng/mL
- 17-OHP, 60 minutes postcosyntropin stimulation: 2.8 ng/mL.

ABDOMINAL USG (ULTRASONOGRAPHY)

Evidence of bilateral enlarged ovaries (volume: right ovary 14.5 mL and left ovary 12.8 mL) with increased echogenicity and multiple peripherally arranged cysts and grade I fatty liver.

Evaluation for metabolic alterations is performed that reveals impaired glucose tolerance (IGT) [after oral glucose tolerance test (OGTT)], and elevated triglyceride (220 mg/dL) and total cholesterol (210 mg/dL), while liver function tests and serum uric acid levels are normal.

DIFFERENTIAL DIAGNOSIS

This patient's history, physical and biochemical features suggesting androgen excess. The most likely etiologies include:

- Polycystic ovarian syndrome (PCOS)
- Nonclassic congenital adrenal hyperplasia (CAH)
- Hyperprolactinemia
- Hypothyroidism
- Cushing's syndrome
- Androgen secreting ovarian or adrenal tumors.

Perimenarchal onset, oligomenorrhea, and an increased LH to FSH ratio are suggestive of PCOS. However, CAH may have identical presentation. Only specific testing would help in establishing the diagnosis. The most prevalent form of CAH is the 21-hydroxylase (*P450c21*) deficiency and this is identified by elevation in plasma concentration of 17-hydroxyprogesterone (17-OHP). A 2 ng/mL threshold for basal 17-OHP plasma concentrations provides 100% sensitivity and 99% specificity for the diagnosis of CAH. This would avoid unnecessary adrenocorticotropic hormone stimulation tests.

In patients with borderline concentrations, levels of 17(OH) progesterone exceeding 10 ng/mL at 60 minutes following injection of 250 μg of cosyntropin accurately diagnoses CAH. Primary hypothyroidism and hyperprolactinemia need to be ruled out on biochemical testing. Women with PCOS should be screened for Cushing syndrome or acromegaly only if there is a clinical suspicion. Tumorous production of testosterone is suspected in those with rapid progression of hyperandrogenism, virilization, or markedly elevated serum testosterone levels. Specific imaging procedures are indicated in such patients to rule out adrenal or ovarian androgen secreting tumor. Given the long-standing nature of the symptoms, mild degree of hirsutism, absence of virilization, and mild hyperandrogenemia in our patient, adrenal or ovarian neoplasm are unlikely.

Hyperandrogenemia is a biochemical marker of PCOS. Elevated androgen levels are seen in 80–90% of women with oligomenorrhea (cycle length >35 days and <8 cycles/year). Vast majority will have elevated free testosterone levels.

Approximately 25–35% of women with PCOS will have elevated levels of DHEAS and this may be the sole abnormality in circulating androgens in approximately 10% of these women.

The number of primary growing follicles in woman with PCOS and anovulation; is sixfold higher than in normal ovulatory women. Antral follicle count is a cornerstone of PCOS diagnosis according to the Rotterdam criteria (ultrasound evidence of 12 or more follicles/ovary essential for diagnosis). However, due to technical advances in imaging, identification of more follicles leads to an artificial increase in the prevalence of polycystic ovaries morphology in normal younger population. A higher threshold of 19 follicles has reported sensitivity and specificity of 81% and 92%, respectively; for the diagnosis of PCOS. Anti-Mullerian hormone (AMH) is produced by the granulosa cells of follicles from the time of initiation of follicle growth. Anti-Mullerian hormone levels essentially reflect the ovarian follicular pool. The expression of AMH is very low in larger antral follicles. Serum AMH levels are two to threefold higher in women with PCOS and correlate well with number of antral follicles, assessed by ultrasound.

Our patient also qualifies for a diagnosis of metabolic syndrome [according to US National Cholesterol Education Program/Adult Treatment Panel III (NCEP/ATP III) criteria] on the basis of obesity (WC 98 cm), hypertension, IGT, and increased serum triglycerides and as such has a high cardiovascular risk.

TREATMENT OPTIONS

The treatment of PCOS is primarily directed at the clinical manifestation, i.e., menstrual irregularity, hirsutism, and infertility. Lifestyle modifications, such as diet and exercise, are considered first-line treatment for women with PCOS. Calorie restriction resulting in weight loss as little as 5% of initial body weight can be effective in regulating menses, restoring ovulatory cycles and achieving pregnancy in obese women with PCOS. The recommended diet for obese women with PCOS is a hypocaloric diet that results in a 500 kcal/day deficit and has reduced glycemic load. This approach has been found to be comparable to or better than treatment with medication. Weight loss in obese women with PCOS also improves hyperandrogenic features.

Medical management of PCOS is aimed at the treatment of metabolic derangements, anovulation, hirsutism, and menstrual irregularity. The main therapeutic emphasis has focused on inhibition of ovarian steroid production and decreased bioavailability through increase in sex hormone-binding globulin (SHBG) levels with the use of oral contraceptive pills (OCPs). The American College of Obstetricians and Gynecologists recommends use of combination low-dose hormonal contraceptive agents for long-term management of menstrual dysfunction. Treatment can be started with a preparation that has a low dose of estrogen and a nonandrogenic progestin. Oral contraceptive pills can induce weight gain and increase blood pressure in some women and raise the risk of thromboembolism in smokers and those with mutations in Factor V Leiden or high levels of lipoprotein(a). Thus, OCPs provide reproductive benefit but confer metabolic risk. In patients who do not have hirsutism but have anovulatory and irregular menstrual cycles, treatment with a single progestin may be attempted as an alternative to OCP. Progestin therapy interrupts the chronic exposure of endometrium to unopposed effects of estrogen. However, this treatment does not decrease androgen excess nor does it provide contraception.

Hirsutism can be effectively treated with low-dose hormonal OCPs. Preparations that have norgestrel and levonorgestrel should be avoided, because of their androgenic activity. Ethinyl estradiol combined with drospirenone has a progestin that acts as an antiandrogen and thus may add antiandrogenic effects. Oral contraceptive pills slow hair growth in 60–100% of women with hyperandrogenemia. Preparations containing cyproterone acetate are very effective in the treatment of more severe hirsutism. If symptoms such as hirsutism are not sufficiently alleviated, OCPs are prescribed in combination with an antiandrogen to block androgen action at the hair follicles. Antiandrogens include spironolactone (an aldosterone-antagonist diuretic), flutamide (an androgen receptor antagonist), and finasteride (a 5α-reductase type-2 inhibitor). In general, the addition of an antiandrogen to OCPs has not appeared to increase the overall treatment benefit. Each of these agents has been shown to reduce hirsutism, and all appear to have equivalent efficacy. Because of its relatively favorable side effect profile and ease of administration, spironolactone (50–100 mg twice daily) is an effective primary therapy for hirsutism in PCOS women, although, liver function tests need to be monitored periodically. Prolonged (>6 months) medical treatment is necessary before effectiveness can be assessed. Pregnancy should be excluded before therapy with oral contraceptives or androgen-blocking agents is started.

Physical approaches to remove unwanted hair, including electrolysis and laser treatments, may be acceptable to many patients. Topical treatment with eflornithine hydrochloride, an inhibitor of ornithine decarboxylase, limits cell division and has been shown to be effective for decreasing the development of new unwanted facial hair.

The use of insulin-sensitizing drugs to improve insulin sensitivity is associated with a reduction in circulating androgen levels, as well as improvement in both the ovulation rate and glucose tolerance. Metformin can be considered in women with PCOS who are insulin resistant and therefore at risk of developing cardiovascular disease (CVD), even in women without type-2 diabetes. Clinical trials have shown that metformin can effectively reduce androgen levels, improve insulin sensitivity, and facilitate weight loss in patients with PCOS as early as adolescence. A long-term study suggested that metformin continued to improve the metabolic profile of women with PCOS over a 36 month treatment course, particularly improving circulating high-density lipoprotein cholesterol, diastolic blood pressure, and body mass index. Given the favorable effect of metformin on lipid profile and progression to diabetes in selected populations, metformin therapy offers many advantages and should be considered, either alone or in combination with other agents, as first-line therapy when metabolic abnormalities are significant. In combination with OCP, metformin may limit weight gain, reduce fasting insulin and glucose levels, improve glucose tolerance, and attenuate the estrogen-dependent rise in plasma triglycerides.

Polycystic ovarian syndrome is a cause of infertility because these women have oligomenorrhea or amenorrhea and also because the menstrual cycles may be anovulatory. Clomiphene citrate (CC) is the first-line treatment for ovulation induction in anovulatory women with PCOS. It is believed that CC acts as an antiestrogen at the hypothalamic level and blocks the negative feedback by estradiol, resulting in increased secretion of FSH. The ovulation rate, conception rate, and live birth rate achieved with CC exceed the respective rates of other modalities used. Treatment is initiated at a dose of 50 mg daily (maximum recommended dose is 150 mg daily) for 5 days and is started 2–5 days after a spontaneous cycle or progesterone-induced withdrawal bleeding. CC treatment is generally limited to 6 ovulatory cycles (may be increased to 12 cycles) and if fertility does not occur, the women is considered to be clomiphene resistant. Ovarian hyperstimulation syndrome is a rare complication.

Metformin, because of its effect on insulin resistance and resulting hyperandrogenemia, has been used for ovulation induction in PCOS women. Earlier studies showed beneficial effects, but recent trials suggest that it is inferior to CC. Although ovulation and pregnancy rates were improved (compared with clomiphene alone) when metformin was used as an adjunct to clomiphene treatment, the live birth rate was unaffected by the addition of metformin. Currently, the use of metformin is limited to those anovulatory PCOS women who have metabolic abnormalities (glucose intolerance), BMI >35 kg/m^2, and resistance to CC. Other insulin-sensitizing agents like thiazolidinediones have been shown to be effective in improving the rate of ovulation (and hyperandrogenemia) in women with PCOS. However, because of their adverse side effects, the consensus is that such medication should be avoided in management of women who are hoping to conceive or who are at risk of pregnancy.

Second-line treatment to induce ovulation in PCOS is low-dose gonadotropin therapy, using human menopausal gonadotropins (hMG) or recombinant FSH (rFSH). Gonadotropin therapy carries a risk of multiple pregnancies and hyperstimulation syndrome.

Surgical approach in the form of bilateral wedge resection has been used to induce ovulation since the early description of PCOS. It is believed that partial destruction of ovarian stroma results in decrease in intraovarian androgens that stimulates FSH release. Recently, laparoscopic procedure like ovarian drilling is performed to improve ovulation and pregnancy rates in women who are resistant to CC treatment. Ovarian drilling is performed with a unipolar electrode that punches four to six holes in each ovary. Adverse effects include hemorrhage, adhesion formation, and ovarian atrophy. Another surgical procedure available is electrocautery (diathermy).

If pregnancy is not achieved by any of the treatments described above, the method of choice is in vitro fertilization (IVF). In IVF is performed by controlled ovarian hyperstimulation with higher doses of rFSH or hMG.

The patient discussed in the case history was counseled about life-style changes including diet modifications and an exercise protocol was suggested. In addition, metformin (500 mg starting dose, increased to 500 mg bid subsequently) was prescribed along with OCPs (ethinyl estradiol plus progestin). Over next 4–6 months, the patient reduced her weight and showed a significant improvement in her hyperandrogenism and metabolic profile.

DISCUSSION

Polycystic ovarian syndrome is a complex and heterogeneous clinical condition characterized by hyperandrogenism and chronic oligoanovulation that may or may not be accompanied by a polycystic ovary. Polycystic ovarian syndrome is one of the most common endocrine disorders reported in approximately 5–10% (upto 20% in some studies using Rotterdam criteria) women of childbearing age and it has both reproductive and metabolic implications. Polycystic ovarian syndrome is associated with an increased incidence of CVD risk factors, including an increased prevalence of subclinical atherosclerosis, dyslipidemia and abnormal glucose regulation. Obesity and insulin resistance are closely linked to the development of PCOS and its clinical features, and the current obesity epidemic suggests the prevalence of PCOS will rise in future.

Diagnosis of Polycystic Ovarian Syndrome

In 1935, Irving Stein and Michael Leventhal observed an association between amenorrhea, hirsutism, and polycystic ovaries (PCO) and described clinical, macroscopic characteristics, and histological features of PCOS for the first time. Different diagnostic criteria have been used for the diagnosis of PCOS. In 1990, a conference sponsored by the US National Institute of Health (NIH) put forward recommendations concerning diagnostic criteria for PCOS, sometimes referred to as "classical PCOS," which included:

- Oligo-ovulation or anovulation manifested by oligomenorrhea or amenorrhea
- Hyperandrogenism (clinical evidence of androgen excess) or hyperandrogenemia (biochemical evidence of androgen excess)
- Exclusion of other disorders that can result in menstrual irregularity and hyperandrogenism.

However after 1990, it became apparent, especially in the infertility setting that many women present with ovarian dysfunction and polycystic ovaries on ultrasound, but without clinical evidence of androgen excess. In 2003, a consensus group, with representatives from the European Society for Human Reproduction and Embryology (ESHRE) and the American Society for Reproductive Medicine (ASRM), modified the criteria to include transvaginal ultrasound evaluation of the ovaries. The 2003, Rotterdam

(ESHRE/ASRM) consensus workshop recommended that after exclusion of secondary causes at least two of the following three features are required for PCOS to be diagnosed after exclusion:

- Oligo-ovulation or anovulation manifested as oligomenorrhea or amenorrhea
- Hyperandrogenism (clinical evidence of androgen excess) or hyperandrogenemia (biochemical evidence of androgen excess)
- Polycystic ovaries (as defined on ultrasonography)
- The use of the Rotterdam criteria had two major consequences: (1) PCOS prevalence increased substantially, from 6–8% to 12–20%; and (2) different PCOS phenotypes were introduced, which were subsequently named classic (characterized by hyperandrogenism and oligoanovulation, with or without PCO morphology, and corresponding to the previous NIH definition), ovulatory (hyperandrogenism and PCO), and normoandrogenic (oligoanovulation and PCO).

During transition through puberty, adolescents commonly have symptoms mimicking all of the diagnostic criteria for PCOS. In adolescents with normal menses, a high prevalence of characteristic polycystic ovaries can be found in otherwise asymptomatic girls, suggesting that the occurrence of this finding is high in the adolescent population. These considerations have led to the suggestion that all three elements of the Rotterdam criteria should be present in teenagers to make the diagnosis of PCOS. To accommodate currently available data and arrive at an evidence-based definition for PCOS, the Androgen Excess and PCOS Society (AE-PCOS) published a position statement in 2006 and its criteria in 2009 emphasizing that, in the society's opinion, PCOS should be considered a disorder of androgen excess, as defined by the following:

- Clinical/biochemical evidence of hyperandrogenism
- Evidence of ovarian dysfunction (oligo-ovulation and/or polycystic ovaries)
- Exclusion of related disorders.

In the AE-PCOS criteria, hyperandrogenism was defined as biochemical (total testosterone >55 ng/mL) or clinical (Ferriman–Gallwey score >8), irregular menses were defined as menses less than nine times/year, and polycystic appearing ovaries were defined as either ovary having a volume of >10 cm^3 on abdominal or transvaginal ultrasound (Table 12.1).

In all these three definitions, hyperandrogenism is defined as clinical and/or biochemical hyperandrogenism. In addition, all these three definitions require the exclusion of other disorders that could mimic PCOS, such as

TABLE 12.1: Diagnostic criteria for polycystic ovarian syndrome

	NIH	ESHRE/ASRM	AE-PCOS
Hyperandrogenism	+	±	+
Oligoanovulation	+	±	±
PCO ultrasound	-	±	±

PCO, Polycystic ovaries; AE-PCOS, Androgen Excess and PCOS Society; NIH, National Institutes of Health; ESHRE, Europian Society for Human Reproduction and Embryology; ASRM, American Society for Reproductive Medicine.

hyperprolactinemia, nonclassical CAH, androgen-secreting tumors, and Cushing's syndrome.

Depending on which criteria are used, the prevalence of PCOS differs in the same population. For example, the diagnostic criteria according to AE-PCOS exclude women without hyperandrogenic symptoms, thus entailing a lower prevalence than the ESHRE/ASRM criteria. Conversely, the AE-PCOS criteria will result in a slightly higher prevalence than the NIH criteria, in which oligoanovulation is only assessed by reports on menstrual disturbances and not by ultrasound features.

In addition to the plausible differences in prevalence rates, it has been suggested that the different criteria may be associated with different metabolic disturbances. For instance, the ESHRE/ASRM criteria will, in addition to women with classical PCOS (i.e. PCOS diagnosed according to NIH criteria), include the PCOS phenotype with oligomenorrhea and polycystic ovaries. This PCOS phenotype is associated with a slightly lower risk for obesity, insulin resistance, and hypertension and possibly, fewer cardiovascular complications.

Pathophysiology of Polycystic Ovarian Syndrome

The pathogenesis of PCOS is multifactorial. The genetic predisposition for PCOS has been evaluated and a familiar clustering is indicated with higher androgen levels, increased prevalence of insulin resistance, and more often CVD in first-degree relatives. The genetic contribution for symptom development in individual subjects is difficult to ascertain although 35% of mothers and 40% of sisters of women with PCOS also display characteristics of the syndrome. Twin studies have shown heritability of 79% for PCOS with a correlation of 0.71 between monozygotic twins and 0.38 between dizygotic twins. Several genetic loci have been proposed to account for the PCOS phenotype. These include *CYP11A1*, the insulin gene, and the fibrillin-3 gene. The lack of a clear-cut phenotype precludes genetic studies of PCOS.

Hyperandrogenism in women with PCOS is considered a consequence of abdominal obesity, insulin resistance and/or resulting hyperinsulinemia, but may also be a contributing factor to the insulin resistance, and abdominal adiposity displayed by patients. The interplay between hyperandrogenism and insulin resistance has led to the suggestion that PCOS and its metabolic comorbidities could be explained by the existence of a "vicious circle," whereby a chronic androgen excess of ovarian and/or adrenal origin results in abdominal adiposity in affected women. Conversely, abdominal adiposity, through insulin resistance and hyperinsulinism, favors further hyperandrogenism through different pathways including the ovaries, hepatic SHBG synthesis, and possibly the pituitary and adrenals. Increased LH secretion by the pituitary gland is consistently demonstrated. It is not clear if this is a primary defect in the GnRH pulse generator or if this is a secondary phenomenon. Increased LH stimulation to the theca cells drives increased androgen production.

There is general agreement that obese women with PCOS are insulin resistant, but some groups of lean affected women may have normal insulin sensitivity. The mechanism of insulin resistance in PCOS remains obscure. There is postreceptor signaling defect that appears to be specific to certain signaling pathways. This selective insulin resistance is illustrated importantly in the ovary, in which the effect of insulin on steroid production remains unimpaired, whereas the metabolic actions of insulin (on glucose uptake and metabolism) are partially inhibited. This ability of the ovarian steroidogenic pathways to "read" insulin in the face of hyperinsulinemia has considerable clinical significance. Insulin acts, along with increased LH secretion, to enhance androgen production from the ovary. Insulin also inhibits hepatic production of SHBG.

Clinical Features of Polycystic Ovarian Syndrome

Most women diagnosed with PCOS in the gynecologic setting, present with symptoms of oligomenorrhea or amenorrhea and seek medical care primarily because they fear their menstrual disturbance may impair future or present fertility. Other reasons for seeking medical care include hirsutism, manifest infertility, and anovulatory menometrorrhagia. Most women are diagnosed after the age of 18–20 years, as hyperandrogenism and menstrual disturbances are considered common symptoms during normal adolescence.

Menstrual Abnormalities

Patients with PCOS have abnormal menstrual patterns attributed to chronic anovulation. Some women have oligomenorrhea (i.e. menstrual bleeding that occurs at intervals of 35 days to 6 months, with <9 menstrual periods/year) or secondary amenorrhea (an absence of menstruation for 6 months). Dysfunctional uterine bleeding and infertility are the other consequences of anovulatory menstrual cycles. The menstrual irregularities in PCOS usually present around the time of menarche. Amenorrheic women with PCOS usually have the most severe hyperandrogenism as compared with women presenting with oligomenorrhea or regular menstrual cycles. Menstrual cycles in women with PCOS become more regular as they approach menopause.

Irregular menses are commonly present during the first few years after menarche. As many as 85% of menstrual cycles are anovulatory during the first year after menarche, and up to 59% are still anovulatory during the third year after menarche. By 2 years postmenarche, menstrual cycles are normal in the majority of adolescents. Based on these findings, some experts suggest that the diagnosis of PCOS should be deferred during the first 2 years after menarche.

Hyperandrogenism

Hyperandrogenism is the most common clinical sign of PCOS and clinically manifests as excess terminal body hair in a male distribution pattern. Hair is commonly seen on the upper lip, on the chin, around the nipples, and along the linea alba of the lower abdomen. Some patients have acne and/or male-pattern hair loss (androgenic alopecia). Hirsutism is a good marker for hyperandrogenism even when considering ethnic differences and systemic factors such as obesity. Hirsutism is present in approximately 70% of women with PCOS, but hyperandrogenemia should be evaluated biochemically in all women suspected of having PCOS. Acne and alopecia are not commonly associated with hyperandrogenemia and therefore should not be regarded as evidence of hyperandrogenemia. Other signs of hyperandrogenism (e.g. clitoromegaly, increased muscle mass, and voice deepening) are more characteristic of an extreme form of PCOS termed hyperthecosis. These signs and symptoms could also be consistent with androgen-producing tumors, exogenous androgen administration, or virilizing CAH.

The modified Ferriman–Gallwey scoring system has been designed to assess the severity of hirsutism. The masculine pattern of body hair growth is described in four degrees on 11 different body places; the upper lip, chin, chest, upper back, lower back, upper abdomen, lower abdomen, arm, forearm, thigh, and buttocks. Although often used in scientific reports on PCOS, the Ferriman–Gallwey score is hampered by the large inter-rater variability and also by the fact that many women have treated themselves prior to clinical evaluation.

Hyperandrogenemia is the biochemical hallmark of PCOS. Elevated circulating androgen levels are observed in 80–90% of women with oligomenorrhea. Elevated total testosterone is the most direct evidence for androgen excess. As approximately 80% of testosterone is bound to SHBG, 19% to albumin, and only 1% of testosterone is free and biologically available and active; total testosterone may not be sufficient for evaluation of androgen status in women. The calculation of the free androgen index from testosterone and SHBG is widely used for assessment of biochemical hyperandrogenism. Free androgen index is affected by circulating levels of SHBG and testosterone, but correlates relatively well with the more costly equilibrium dialysis method. Free testosterone is possible to measure with a direct immunoassay method but the assay only retrieves 20–60% of the levels compared with the equilibrium dialysis method, the gold standard free testosterone analysis.

Although, PCOS is considered a part of the spectrum of normogonadotropic normoestrogenic anovulation, serum LH concentrations and the LH to FSH ratio are frequently elevated (ratio > 2:1) in affected women. FSH levels are normal to slightly suppressed. However, gonadotropin levels have never been included in any of the diagnostic criteria for PCOS because the characteristic derangements can escape detection on random blood samples because of the pulsatile nature of LH release.

Infertility

A subset of women with PCOS is subfertile which is mostly due to oligoanovulation and metabolic alterations. Conception may take longer than in other women. Women, with PCOS may exhibit reduced developmental competence of the oocyte. Ovarian hyperandrogenism and hyperinsulinemia may promote premature granulosa cell luteinization and paracrine dysregulation of growth factors may disrupt the intrafollicular environment.

Miscarriage rates among women with PCOS are believed to be increased threefold compared with normal fertile women. Endometrial abnormalities, poor quality of oocytes, obesity, and other intrinsic factors have been suggested to affect implantation and increase the risk for miscarriage. Insulin resistance, obesity, and hyperandrogenism, common in PCOS women, are associated with increased risk of preeclampsia, gestational diabetes, preterm birth, and stillbirth. In women with PCOS, there is a higher incidence of gestational diabetes (GDM) (40–50%) and associated fetal macrosomia, and birth of small-for-gestational-age babies (10–15%).

Metabolic Consequences of Polycystic Ovarian Syndrome

Polycystic ovarian syndrome is associated with metabolic disturbances such as insulin resistance and hyperinsulinism, type-2 diabetes, dyslipidemia, and possibly cardiovascular disease (CVD). Studies over the past two decades have indicated that insulin resistance is a pathogenic characteristic feature of the PCOS. Both lean and obese women with PCOS are generally more insulin resistant than normal women matched for total and free body mass. Insulin resistance is most prevalent and severe in those with the classic NIH PCOS phenotype involving hyperandrogenism and chronic anovulation. Increased insulin resistance appears a crucial mechanism behind the association of PCOS and metabolic disturbances and is a common feature in PCOS and the metabolic syndrome (MetS).

The MetS is a cluster of metabolic disturbances that increases the risk of CVD and diabetes. According to a scientific statement of the American Heart Association and the NCEP/ATP III, the metabolic syndrome is present if three of following five criteria are fulfilled: elevated waist circumference, elevated triglycerides, reduced high-density lipoprotein (HDL) cholesterol, elevated blood pressure, and elevated fasting glucose. Prevalence of the MetS in PCOS women vary between 11% and 47.3% in various studies.

There is considerable ethnic variation in the expression of PCOS, including the prevalence and severity of obesity, metabolic disturbances, and their correlates. Asian women are generally shorter, have a lower BMI, and a milder hyperandrogenic phenotype. South Asians in particular have a high prevalence of MetS and are at risk for type-2 diabetes, with central obesity more than BMI reflecting their metabolic risk. There is a strikingly high prevalence of hirsutism among women of Middle Eastern and Mediterranean origin. Nevertheless, abnormal glucose tolerance in Southern and Eastern Europeans is far less common than in South Asians and Hispanics. There is widespread variability in the prevalence of overweight (BMI 25–30 kg/m^2) and obese (BMI >30 kg/m^2) women in PCOS populations across different countries. The highest prevalence of obesity is reported in studies conducted in the United States and Australia, with 61–76% of women with PCOS considered obese.

Polycystic ovarian syndrome is associated with increased risk of IGT, GDM, and type-2 diabetes. Biochemical screening in the form of an OGTT should be performed in the following conditions: hyperandrogenism with anovulation, acanthosis nigricans, obesity (BMI >30 kg/m^2, or >25 kg/m^2 in Asian populations), in women with a family history of T2D or GDM. Risk of IGT or diabetes is highest in women who have both oligo-ovulation or anovulation and hyperandrogenism.

As PCOS women tend to have increased abdominal fat, they are more predisposed to dyslipidemia, as the centrally located adipocytes seem to exert an adverse effect on blood lipids. Various studies have shown that about 70% of PCOS women have abnormal serum lipid levels and dyslipidemia might be the most common metabolic abnormality in PCOS. The dyslipidemia in PCOS includes elevated levels of LDL and triglycerides and decreased levels of HDL.

Quality of Life and Mental Health in PCOS

Polycystic ovarian syndrome is not only associated with metabolic consequences and reduced fertility, but may also influence the quality of life and mental health of affected women. Patients with PCOS are at-risk group for psychological and behavioral disorders and reduced quality of life (QOL). Although most research in the field of mental health and PCOS is devoted to the psychological consequences of infertility, other symptom of PCOS may, individually or in concert, negatively affect QOL, and mental health of women with PCOS. Independent of obesity/overweight, clinical depression, and depressive symptoms appear to be more common among PCOS women than in weight matched controls. Likewise, anxiety symptoms including phobic symptoms appear to be more common among PCOS patients. Needless to say, clinical depression is important to identify in PCOS patients, not only because of the specific disease burden associated with major depression, but also because reduced motivation is a common feature of depression. Reduced motivation; in turn, may negatively impact the success of weight-reducing therapies.

Cancer Risk in Polycystic Ovarian Syndrome

Polycystic ovarian syndrome may be associated with increased risk of the development of cancer of the endometrium, ovary, and/or breast; either directly or mediated by its associated reproductive-metabolic alterations. A recent meta-analysis showed an almost three times higher risk of developing endometrial cancer for PCOS women (OR: 2.70; 95% CI: 1.00–7.29) compared to women without PCOS. The mechanism behind endometrial cancer in PCOS that has been discussed is the unopposed stimulation by estrogens of the endometrium, which can cause endometrial hyperplasia with increased risk of atypia and eventually endometrial cancer. Most endometrial cancers are well differentiated and have a good prognosis.

CONCLUSION

Polycystic ovarian syndrome is a heterogeneous disorder of functional androgen excess, detectable either by laboratory analysis, or by clinical examination. Polycystic ovarian syndrome remains a diagnosis of exclusion and it is essential to exclude other potential etiologies that can present with hyperandrogenism. The prevalence of PCOS will depend to a degree on the criteria used to define this disorder. An increased awareness of PCOS in the general population and the medical communities in recent years has led to greater understanding of the long-term associations of this disorder. The syndrome presents multiple challenges to the patients and the providers at different stages of life including hirsutism, menstrual disturbances, infertility, obesity, and metabolic disturbances. A worrisome complication in women with PCOS who have prolonged periods of amenorrhea is endometrial carcinoma. Insulin resistance is believed to be central to the pathogenesis of this syndrome in a large subset of women who are overweight/obese. The availability and use of multiple treatment modalities and medications attests the lack of a uniformly effective treatment. This syndrome is likely to stay as the focus of intense research on reproductive health in women.

SUGGESTED READINGS

1. Azziz R, Carmina E, Dewailly D, et al. Task Force on the Phenotype of the Polycystic Ovary Syndrome of the Androgen Excess and PCOS Society. The Androgen Excess and PCOS Society criteria for the polycystic ovary syndrome: the complete task force report. Fertil Steril. 2009;91:456-88.
2. Diamanti-Kandarakis E, Dunaif A. Insulin resistance and the polycystic ovary syndrome revisited: an update on mechanisms and implications. Endocr Rev. 2012;33:981-1030.
3. The Rotterdam ESHRE/ASRM-Sponsored PCOS Consensus Workshop Group. Revised 2003 consensus on diagnostic criteria and long-term health risks related to polycystic ovary syndrome. Fertil Steril. 2004;81:19-25.

CHAPTER

13

Addison's Disease/ Adrenal Crisis

Narendra Kotwal

CASE PRESENTATION

A 42-year-old lady presented with complaints of generalized weakness, fatigue, frequent retching, nausea with vomiting, and diarrhea of one year duration. She received symptomatic treatment for dyspepsia and vomiting in form of proton pump inhibitors and prokinetic agents. Earlier a dermatologist diagnosed her as a case of limited scleroderma and administered pulse therapy of dexamethasone and penicillamine, which improved her symptoms. However, after discontinuation of dexamethasone therapy, she had recurrence of her previous symptoms. She was referred to psychiatrist for persistent nonspecific symptoms and diagnosed as a case of anxiety neurosis and treated with benzodiazepines and antidepressants. She was subsequently referred to rheumatologist at tertiary hospital for nonspecific joint pains. Suspecting Addison's disease, rheumatologist referred her to endocrinologist for evaluation and management. When seen in endocrine clinic she reported having anorexia, nausea for last 18 months; increased skin pigmentation particularly over sun exposed areas, vomiting and diarrhea on and off for last 1 year; and weight loss of around 10 kg over last 6 months. She also reported postural giddiness and salt craving. There was no history of cough, evening rise of fever, night sweats. No history of hypopigmented spots over body, chronic mucocutaneous candidiasis, or spontaneous carpopedal spasms. No hypometabolic symptoms, osmotic symptoms. No history suggestive of Reynaud's phenomenon. There was no past history of tuberculosis, diabetes mellitus, hypertension, thyroid disease, Jaundice, or blood transfusion. She denied any history of chronic steroid intake. No family history of tuberculosis, thyroid disease, or similar illness. She had normal menstrual history with menstrual cycle of 29 days. No history of recurrent miscarriage. On examination, her blood pressure was 84/60 mmHg supine and 72/50 mmHg after standing for 3 minutes. Her heart rate was 108 beats/minute, regular, low volume; thread pulse without any radio radial or radio femoral delay. Also diffuse hyperpigmentation, more over sun exposed areas, nipples, gums, and areas of friction were noted. Loss of axillary and pubic hair was also noted. No hypopigmented spots were noted. Remainder of systemic examination was otherwise normal.

DIFFERENTIAL DIAGNOSIS

- Hypercalcemia/hyperparathyroidism (D/D for anorexia and vomiting)
- Hypopituitarism (D/D for fatigue)
- Chemoradiotherapy (D/D for anorexia and vomiting)
- Anorexia nervosa and depression (D/D for anorexia, vomiting)
- Chronic kidney disease (D/D for fatigue, nausea)
- Chronic liver failure (D/D for fatigue, nausea, anorexia)
- Chronic heart disease (D/D for fatigue)
- Ca stomach/gastric ulcer (D/D fatigue, weight loss, anorexia)
- HIV/AIDS infection.

EVALUATION

She was provisionally diagnosed as a case of adrenal crisis. Samples were drawn for routine hematological and biochemical profile including measurement of serum cortisol and adrenocorticotropic hormone (ACTH). Patient was treated with intravenous normal saline with dextrose and hydrocortisone infusion, pending results of investigations. Her blood pressure improved rapidly and there was marked symptomatic improvement. She had evidence of microcytic hypochromic anemia with low serum ferritin levels. Her blood urea nitrogen was 37 mg/dL (normal range: 10–15 mg/dL) and serum creatinine was 0.9 mg/dL (normal range: 0.4–1.4 mg/dL). She had hyponatremia (serum Na: 118 meq/L). Her Basal cortisol was 2.6 µg/dL (normal range: 5–24 µg/dL), with concurrent plasma ACTH of 754 pg/mL (normal range: 10–72 pg/mL). Once her condition stabilized, patient underwent a standard ACTH stimulation test confirming primary adrenal insufficiency (basal/stimulated cortisol: 0.4/1.4 µg/dL). Etiological workup revealed positive mantoux's test (induration of 22 mm at 72 hours). Computed tomography (CT) scan adrenal revealed bilateral adrenal enlargement with calcification. In view of these findings primary adrenal insufficiency was ascribed to tubercular adrenalitis. She was treated with hydrocortisone given three times daily (10-5-5 mg) and fludrocortisone 0.1 mg once daily. Additionally, she was placed on antituberculosis therapy (ATT). On starting ATT, dose of hydrocortisone was increased. Also she was educated about stress dosing of hydrocortisone. She responded favorably to treatment.

MANAGEMENT

Patients with primary adrenal insufficiency require chronic glucocorticoid and mineralocorticoid replacement. Those in adrenal crisis should be immediately started on hydrocortisone and normal saline with dextrose. Our patient was started on glucocorticoid and mineralocorticoid replacement therapy (hydrocortisone replacement at 10 mg/m^2 is given in three divided doses). The two thirds of the dose were given in the morning and the remaining dose was given in the afternoon and early evening. This is to mimic dynamic of normal plasma cortisol. Other long acting steroids like dexamethasone and prednisolone are not preferred, as they cannot mimic normal contour of glucocorticoid secretion. Additionally, she also received fludrocortisone replacement at the dosage of 100 µg daily. Patient had bilateral enlarged adrenal glands with calcification (various causes of bilateral adrenal enlargement are mentioned in Table 13.1). In India, the commonest cause of primary adrenal insufficiency is tubercular adrenalitis and in the western world it is autoimmune adrenalitis. Patient also had bilateral calcification of adrenal glands (often seen in patients with adrenal tuberculosis). On initiation of ATT, hydrocortisone doses were increased since rifampicin is an enzyme inducer, and enhances clearance of hydrocortisone. The patient responded well to ATT. Patient is under follow-up and is doing well.

DISCUSSION

In 1855, Thomas Addison first described a disease characterized by salt wasting and hyperpigmentation as the result of adrenal gland destruction, and consequent adrenal insufficiency. Addison was a medical student in Edinburgh and went on to be one of the three "giants" of Guys hospital (together with Richard Bright and Thomas Hodgkin).

Addison's disease remained a fatal condition till the achievement of the synthesis of cortisone in 1949 (*Kendell, Sarett, and Reichstein*) and its introduction into therapeutic use in the early 1950s. There are two types of

TABLE 13.1: Causes of bilateral adrenal enlargement

• Tuberculosis	• Histoplasmosis
• Pheochromocytoma—familial/children	• Cryptococcosis
• Metastasis to adrenal	• Amyloidosis
• Congenital adrenal hyperplasia	• Adrenal hemorrhage
• Cushing's disease	• Disseminated NHL
• Ectopic secretion of CRH, ACTH	• Primary adrenal lymphoma

ACTH, adrenocorticotropic hormone; CRH, corticotropin hormone; NHL, non-Hodgkin lymphoma.

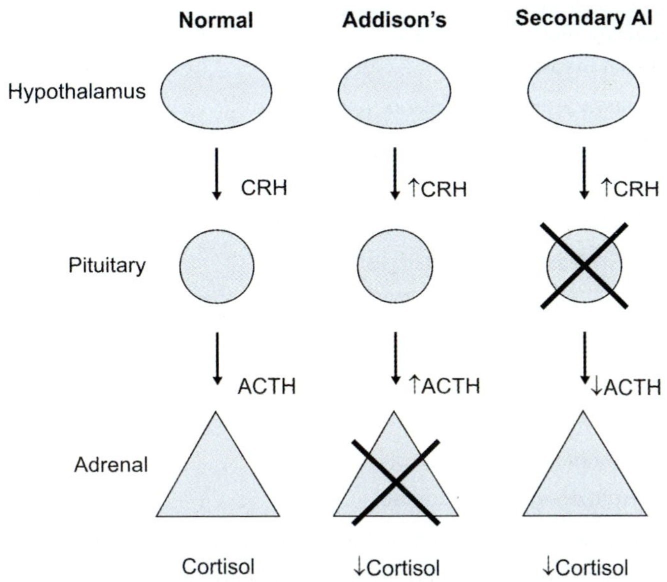

CRH, corticotropin releasing hormone; ACTH, adrenocorticotropic hormone; AI, adrenal insufficiency.

Figure 13.1: Primary and secondary adrenal insufficiency

adrenal insufficiency: primary and secondary (Fig. 13.1). Primary adrenal insufficiency has a prevalence of 93–140 per million and an incidence of 4·7–6·2 per million in white populations. Addison's disease usually peaks in the fourth decade of life, with women more frequently affected than men. Secondary adrenal insufficiency has an estimated prevalence of 150–280 per million, and also affects women more frequently than men. Age at diagnosis peaks in the sixth decade of life. Exogenous glucocorticoid administration is thought to be the most common cause of secondary adrenal insufficiency, since chronic administration of steroids induces atrophy of pituitary corticotroph cells. In active tuberculosis, the incidence of adrenal involvement is 5%. In developed countries, 80–90% of patients with primary adrenal insufficiency have autoimmune adrenalitis, which can arise as isolated (40%; slight male preponderance) or as part of an autoimmune polyendocrine syndrome (APS) (60%; female preponderance). The causes of primary adrenal insufficiency are mentioned in Table 13.2.

Autoimmune polyendocrine syndrome type 1, also termed autoimmune polyendocrinopathy-candidiasis-ectodermal dystrophy (APECED), arises in up to 15% of patients with autoimmune adrenalitis. It is characterized by adrenal insufficiency, hypoparathyroidism, and chronic mucocutaneous candidiasis with onset during childhood. APECED is caused by mutations

TABLE 13.2: Causes of adrenal insufficiency

Primary adrenal insufficiency

- Anatomic damage to adrenal gland
  - "Idiopathic" atrophy (autoimmune)
  - Adrenoleukodystrophy
  - Infections (tuberculosis, fungal, viral in AIDS)
  - Metastases/invasion (neoplastic, sarcoidosis)
  - Hemorrhage (anticoagulants, Waterhouse–Friderichsen syndrome)
  - Infarction (antiphospholipid syndrome)
  - Surgery
- Reduced steroid biosynthesis
  - CAH (congenital adrenal hyperplasia)
  - Use of cytotoxic agents (mitotane)
  - Use of enzyme inhibitors (aminoglutethimide, ketoconazole, metapyrone)
- ACTH receptor gene mutation (Allgrove' syndrome also known as triple A syndrome: **a**drenal insufficiency, **a**lacrima, and **a**chalasia)
- Adrenal hypoplasia congenital (mutation in *DAX1* gene)
- ACTH blocking antibodies

Secondary adrenal insufficiency

- Hypopituitarism due hypothalamic-pituitary disease
  - Congenital
  - Acquired (Sheehan's syndrome/hemorrhage, hypophysitis, trauma, irradiation, surgery, neoplasm, infiltration—sarcoidosis, isolated ACTH deficiency)
- Suppression of HPA axis by exogenous or endogenous steroids

in the autoimmune regulator gene and it is inherited in an autosomal recessive fashion. Adrenal insufficiency is also seen in APS 2. APS type 2 is the most frequently seen APS and comprises Addison's disease, primary hypothyroidism, primary hypogonadism, type-1 diabetes, pernicious anemia, and vitiligo. The inheritance of APS 2 (Schmidt's syndrome) is autosomal dominant with incomplete penetrance and shows a strong association with HLA-DR3 and cytotoxic T-lymphocyte-associated protein 4 (CTLA-4). APS 4 is presence of adrenal insufficiency with any autoimmune disorder but without thyroid disease and APS 3 involves autoimmune thyroid disease but not adrenal insufficiency.

The X-linked adrenoleukodystrophy is caused by a mutation in the *ABCD1* gene (normally it encodes a peroxisomal membrane protein—adrenoleukodystrophy protein), leading to accumulation of very-long-chain fatty acids (>24 carbon atoms). Clinically patient presents as a case of adrenal insufficiency and neurological impairment due to white-matter demyelination. The two major forms are cerebral adrenoleukodystrophy (50% of cases; early childhood manifestation; rapid progression) and adrenomyeloneuropathy (35% of cases; onset in early adulthood; slow progression) with restriction of demyelination to spinal cord and peripheral nerves. Adrenal insufficiency can precede the onset of neurological symptoms and is the sole manifestation of disease in 15% of cases. Adrenoleukodystrophy is the most common form of adrenal insufficiency in a child younger than 7 years of age. Other causes of primary adrenal insufficiency, e.g. adrenal infiltration or hemorrhage—are rare. Congenital or neonatal primary adrenal insufficiency accounts for only 1% of all cases.

CLINICAL PRESENTATION

Glucocorticoids are secreted from the adrenal zona fasciculata. It is under the control of hypothalamic corticotropin-releasing hormone (CRH) and pituitary corticotropin (ACTH). The secretion of cortisol shows diurnal pattern with highest concentrations measured early in the morning and lowest concentrations noted around midnight. Mineralocorticoids are produced by the zona glomerulosa. They are mainly under the control of the renin-angiotensin system. Thus, mineralocorticoid secretion is preserved in secondary adrenal insufficiency. Dehydroepiandrosterone secretion by the zona reticularis is also diurnal and is acutely increased by ACTH. Patients with acute adrenal insufficiency/adrenal crisis typically present with severe hypotension or hypovolemic shock, acute abdominal pain, vomiting, and often fever. Such individuals are therefore, sometimes misdiagnosed as having an acute abdomen. In children, adrenal insufficiency (AI) can present as hypoglycemic seizures. Recurrent hypoglycemia in a case of type-1 diabetes can be the first presenting feature of adrenal insufficiency. Hyperpigmentation, due to chronic ACTH and pro-opiomelanocortin related peptides hypersecretion, and weight loss, are indicative of long-standing adrenal insufficiency, while additional symptoms and signs relating to the primary cause of adrenal insufficiency may also be present. Hypotension is the main clinical presenting feature of adrenal crisis due to mineralocorticoid deficiency. It can also occur in patients receiving appropriate doses of glucocorticoid if their mineralocorticoid requirements are not met. However, glucocorticoid deficiency can also contribute to hypotension by decreasing vascular responsiveness to angiotensin II, norepinephrine and other vasoconstrictive hormones, reducing the synthesis of renin substrate, and increasing the production and effects of prostacyclin and other vasodilatory hormones. Chronic adrenal insufficiency usually presents as fatigue, accompanied by lack of stamina, loss of energy, reduced muscle strength, and increased irritability. Also chronic glucocorticoid deficiency leads to weight loss, nausea, and anorexia (anorexia or failure to thrive in children), and can account for muscle and joint pain. Unfortunately, most of the symptoms of chronic AI are nonspecific and there may be a time lag of up to 1 year for diagnosis of Addison's disease in most patients. This is very similar to our patient where she was shunted from psychiatrist to rheumatologist for treatment before being diagnosed as Addison's disease. A very specific sign of Addison's disease is hyperpigmentation, which is most commonly seen in areas of the skin exposed to increased friction—e.g. palmar creases, knuckles, scars, and oral mucosa. Our patient had a similar clinical presentation. It is due to stimulation of skin MC1-receptor by ACTH and other pro-opiomelanocortin-related peptides. The change in the color of the skin can be seen in the photograph of our patient. Laboratory findings in glucocorticoid deficiency can include mild anemia, lymphocytosis, and eosinophilia. Hyponatremia with hyperkalemia are usually the laboratory findings in mineralocorticoid deficiency. Thyrotropin (TSH) release is physiologically inhibited by cortisol. Thus, TSH can be elevated in AI, which returns to normal levels after treatment for AI unless there is a coexisting autoimmune thyroid dysfunction. Also caution should be exercised in patients with both autoimmune thyroid dysfunction and adrenal insufficiency. Initiation of thyroxine prior to steroids in this subset of patients can lead to precipitation of adrenal crisis. AI also leads to dehydroepiandrosterone (DHEA) deficiency. DHEA is a major precursor of sex steroids. Loss of this leads to pronounced androgen deficiency in women and they can present with loss of axillary and pubic hair like in our patient. It can also present as decreased libido in adults and absence of pubarche in children. Also DHEA is known to have potent antidepressant properties. So in spite of adequate glucocorticoid and mineralocorticoid replacement, patients of AI can present with depressive symptoms. Our patient was referred to the psychiatrist for her nonspecific symptoms and diagnosed as a case of anxiety neurosis and was put on benzodiazepines.

LABORATORY DIAGNOSIS

Biochemical features such as hyponatremia, hyperkalemia, hypercalcemia, transient elevations of serum transaminases can be seen. Hypercalcemia can be due to increased intestinal absorption of calcium from the intestine and also increased mobilization of calcium from the bone. Clinical suspicion of the diagnosis should be confirmed with definitive diagnostic tests. A low basal plasma cortisol with concurrent-elevated plasma ACTH is highly suggestive. Basal plasma cortisol and urinary free cortisol levels are often in the low-normal range and cannot be used to exclude the diagnosis. Basal cortisol >14.5 µg/dL excludes adrenal insufficiency. To confirm the diagnosis of adrenal insufficiency ACTH stimulation test should be used. The ACTH stimulation test (short Synacthen test, SST) involves intramuscular or intravenous administration of 250 µg tetracosactin, a synthetic ACTH (1-24) comprising the first 24 amino acids of normally secreted ACTH (1-39). Plasma cortisol levels are measured at 0 and 30 minutes after ACTH administration and a normal response is defined by a peak plasma cortisol level >550 nmol/L (>20 µg/dL). There are various other tests such as the low dose SST, prolonged ACTH stimulation test used primarily to differentiate secondary hypoadrenalism from primary adrenal insufficiency. Insulin tolerance test (ITT) is considered as the gold standard to assess the integrity of the hypothalamic pituitary adrenal (HPA) axis. Insulin tolerance test has to be performed under close supervision and is contraindicated in presence of underlying ischemic heart disease and seizure disorder. However, the cortisol response to hypoglycemia can be reliably predicted by the SST—a safer, cheaper, and quicker test. Usually ITT is reserved if an underlying hypopituitarism is also suspected in the patient. Metapyrone test and CRH tests are the two other tests that can be used to assess the adequacy of HPA axis. Adrenal cortex autoantibodies or antibodies against 21-hydroxylase are present in >80% of patients with recent onset autoimmune adrenalitis. However, some patients may have autoantibodies against other steroidogenic enzymes like P450scc and P450c17.

IMAGING

Adrenal imaging is not indicated in patients with an unequivocal diagnosis of autoimmune adrenalitis or adrenomyeloneuropathy. If infection, hemorrhage, infiltration, or neoplasm is suspected then adrenal CT scan can be obtained. Adrenal tuberculosis presents with bilateral enlarged adrenal glands in the subacute phase with calcifications appearing much later. Our patient had bilateral enlarged adrenal glands with calcifications.

TREATMENT

Currently hydrocortisone is considered as the glucocorticoid of choice for replacement therapy in cases of adrenal insufficiency. A daily oral dose of hydrocortisone of 10-15 mg seems sufficient for replacement, with slightly higher doses for primary than secondary adrenal insufficiency. The current glucocorticoid replacement regimen aims to mimic the physiological diurnal variation of cortisol. However, hydrocortisone results in steep rise of cortisol levels to supraphysiological levels within 2 hours of administration followed by a rapid decline within the next 5–6 hours. In general, glucocorticoid replacement is administered in two or three daily doses, with the first dose on waking, and the last dose approximately 4–6 hours before bed time. Type-1 diabetes patients may need an evening dose to prevent nocturnal hypoglycemia. Prednisolone can be used in selected cases with severe compliance problems, but dexamethasone has no place in replacement therapy for AI. Two slow release preparations of hydrocortisone have been tested in the last few years: Chronocort and Duocort. At higher doses, hydrocortisone also exerts potent mineralocorticoid action, whereas synthetic glucocorticoids only have reduced mineralocorticoid activity (prednisolone) or none at all (dexamethasone), which is an issue of considerable importance for the replacement strategy in patients with primary adrenal insufficiency.

There is no reliable convenient marker for monitoring of the glucocorticoid therapy. Monitoring is based on clinical judgment and looking for signs of over replacement. Weight gain, impaired glucose tolerance, osteoporosis, and hypertension may indicate over replacement and the reverse indicate under replacement. In primary AI patient, levels of plasma adrenocorticotropin (ACTH) are high before administration of hydrocortisone, followed by a quick drop in ACTH levels. Furthermore normalizing ACTH levels often results in Cushingoid appearance, suggesting overreplacement. Hence, ACTH alone cannot be used to monitor adequacy of replacement therapy.

Mineralocorticoids are replaced by oral administration of 9α-fludrocortisone. Mineralocorticoid replacement (only required in primary adrenal insufficiency) consists of oral administration of 0.05–0.2 mg fludrocortisone. The mineralocorticoid activity of this is about 125 times that of hydrocortisone. The adequacy of mineralocorticoid replacement should be assessed by measuring electrolytes, supine and erect blood pressures, and plasma renin activity. In patients who develop primary hypertension, the dose of fludrocortisone may be reduced. With respect to the mineralocorticoid potency, 20 mg of hydrocortisone is equivalent to 0.05 mg fludrocortisone. Mineralocorticoids may be used as glucocorticoid sparing agent as long as no worsening of hypertension and fluid-electrolyte balance occurs.

Dehydroepiandrosterone replacement in a case of primary AI has reported to have an increase in well-being and improved mood. Treatment should be reserved for patients who have a markedly low well-being, despite adequate glucocorticoid and mineralocorticoid replacement. A dose of 25–50 mg to be given once daily in the morning. However, the criteria for dosage replacement of DHEA in elderly in whom a physiological decline with age in DHEA levels occurs, needs to be established.

Adrenal crisis: A state of acute hypoadrenalism accompanied by marked electrolyte and fluid disturbance. Untreated, it can be fatal. In cases of Adrenal crisis, immediate administration of 100 mg hydrocortisone intravenously, followed by 100 mg given every 8 hours with administration of large amounts of normal saline-dextrose (initially 1 L/h) under close cardiac supervision is often lifesaving. A hydrocortisone infusion at 10 Mhs/h can also be chosen as an alternative way of administering glucocorticoid. Precipitating cause must be identified and treated (such as fulminant infection). Once acute emergency has passed, patient can be transitioned to stable oral replacement regimen of glucocorticoid and mineralocorticoid. To prevent adrenal crisis, patients should be educated to double or triple the doses of steroid preparation for the length of the illness or hospitalization (Figs 13.2 to 13.4).

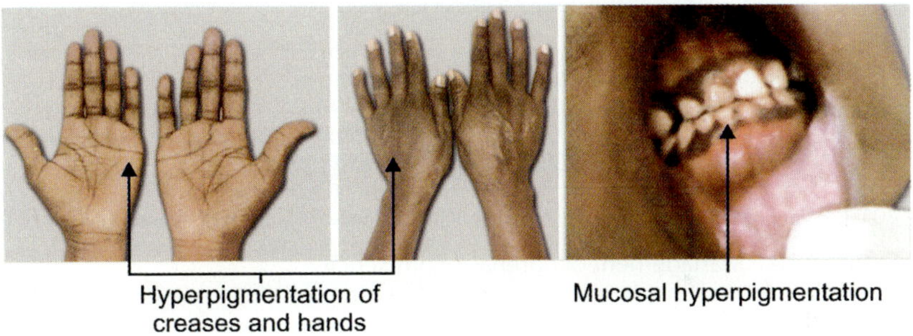

Figure 13.2: Hyperpigmentation of creases and hands and mucosal hyperpigmentation

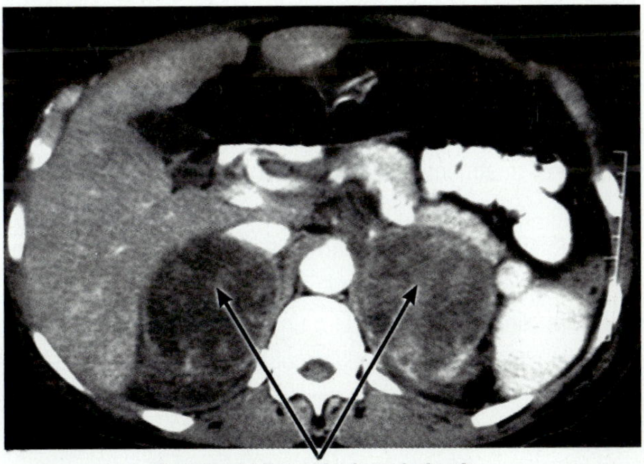

Figure 13.3: Enlarged bilateral adrenal glands

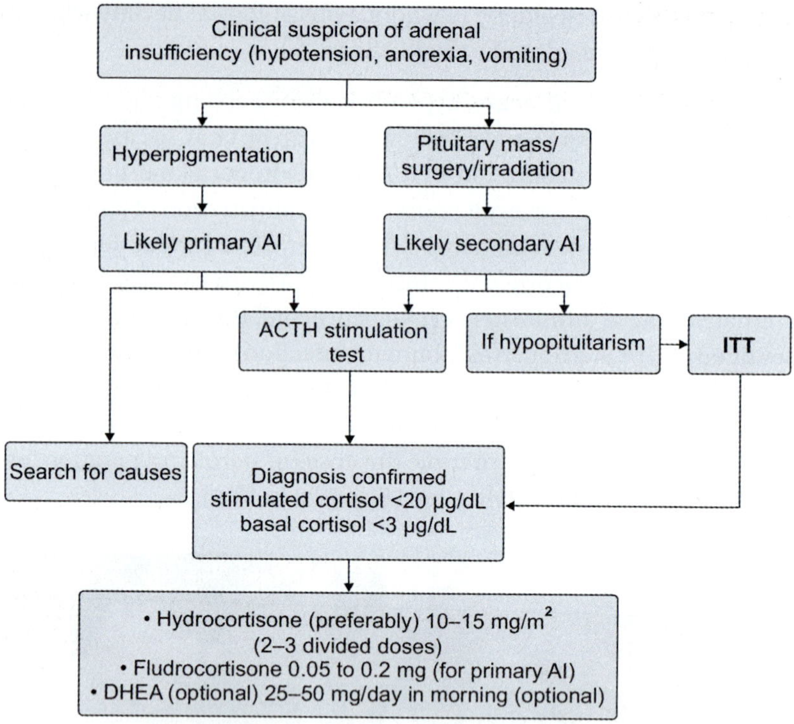

ACTH, adrenocorticotropic hormone; AI, adrenal insufficiency; ITT, insulin tolerance test.

Figure 13.4: Management of adrenal insufficiency

KEY POINTS

- Primary adrenal insufficiency has nonspecific presenting features and a high index of suspicion is necessary for diagnosis
- In India the commonest cause of adrenal insufficiency is tuberculosis
- Treatment should never be delayed and all the necessary samples should be taken prior to initiation of treatment with glucocorticoids
- Cases of secondary adrenal insufficiency can be missed by doing the short synacthen test (SST) especially if done within 4–6 weeks of surgery, as it may take 6 weeks for adrenal glands to atrophy in absence of ACTH
- Patient should be clinically monitored for under or over replacement as no validated measurement for assessing the adequacy of glucocorticoid replacement
- Patient should be educated to double the dosage of glucocorticoid during periods of intercurrent illness for the duration of illness
- If the patient reports feeling of low well-being despite being on adequate glucocorticoid and mineralocorticoid replacement then DHEA replacement should be considered.

SUGGESTED READINGS

1. Arlt W, Allolio B. Adrenal insufficiency. Lancet. 2003;361(9372):1881-93.
2. Arlt W. The approach to the adult with newly diagnosed adrenal insufficiency. J Clin Endocrinol Metab. 2009;94(4):1059-67.
3. Shikama N, Nusspaumer G, Holländer GA. Clearing the AIRE: on the pathophysiological basis of the autoimmune polyendocrinopathy syndrome type-1. Endocrinol Metab Clin North Am. 2009;38(2): 273-88.
4. Stewart P, Krone N. The adrenal cortex. In: Melmed S, Polonsky KS, Larsen PR, Kronenberg HM (Eds), 12th edition. Williams Textbook of Endocrinology. Saunders Elsevier; 2011. pp. 479–544.

CHAPTER

14

Hirsutism

AC Ammini

INTRODUCTION

Hirsutism refers to excess terminal hair in females in areas resembling male pattern of distribution. It is a frustrating experience for women and a complex management problem for clinicians. It is often a clinical indicator of hyperandrogenism and due to conversion of light vellus hair (nonmedullated, short, soft, and lightly pigmented) to dark terminal hair (medullated, stiff, and pigmented) in androgen sensitive body areas.

Hair has a well-defined growth cycle (active growth phase *anagen*; resting phase *telogen*, and shedding phase *catagen*). Hirsutism reflects a response to androgen excess or end-organ super sensitivity to normally circulating androgens. In normal premenopausal women, ovaries, and adrenals contribute equally to circulating testosterone concentrations (about 50% of serum testosterone results from direct secretion by ovaries and adrenals and the remainder is derived from metabolism of androstenedione in peripheral tissue such as fat and skin).

Although testosterone is the most important circulating androgen, it must be converted to dihydrotestosterone (DHT) by enzyme 5á-reductase located in the pilosebaceous unit (PSU) to mediate hirsutism. Androgens are necessary for terminal hair and PSU development. Local production of DHT allows it to serve as the primary androgen mediator of hirsutism.

Clinical severity of hirsutism can be graded with Ferriman–Gallwey score (a semiobjective, semiquantitative scoring of hair growth in nine different skin areas scored from 1 to 4). Ferriman–Gallwey score is usually <8 in healthy women. Other cutaneous conditions associated with androgen excess are androgenetic alopecia, acanthosis nigricans, and acne. Hirsutism must be distinguished from hypertrichosis that refers to generalized hair growth unrelated to androgen excess (commonly seen with phenytoin, cyclosporine, corticosteroids, cetirizine, and citalopram). It should be noted that cutaneous response to androgen excess is genetically determined accounting for different prevalence in different racial/ethnic groups. Women from the Indian subcontinent and Mediterranean countries have higher prevalence compared to those with northern European or East Asian origin.

Clinical evaluation of patients must include a detailed history covering important elements such as age of thelarche (breast development), age of menarche and subsequent menstrual pattern, age of onset, severity of hair growth, and impact on daily life.

CASE PRESENTATION

Ms KP, a 25-year-old female, presented to our endocrine clinic with history of excessive hair growth over face, chest, abdomen, back, arms, and legs over last 18 years duration. She had to remove hair every 3–4 days. She attained menarche at 15 years of age and had irregular menstrual cycles, once every 3–4 months. She was aware of enlarged clitoris from 13 years of age. There was no salt wasting crisis, frequent hospitalization, or failure to thrive. She was the eldest of 4 siblings, from a nonconsanguineous marriage. Her 3 younger siblings were healthy. There was no history of hirsutism, precocious puberty, or infertility in the family.

Her height, weight, and body mass index were 147 cm, 48 kg, and 22.21 kg/m^2. Her blood pressure was 106/82 mmHg and HR 89/min. There was no acanthosis, skin tags, goiter, or Cushingoid features. She had temporal recession of hair, black thick hair over the upper lip, chin and sideburns, and acne Ferriman-Gallwey score was 20 (Fig. 14.1). She had marked clitoromegaly, separate urethral and vaginal opening, and posterior labial fusion. Breast was Tanner grade 2. Systemic examination was normal.

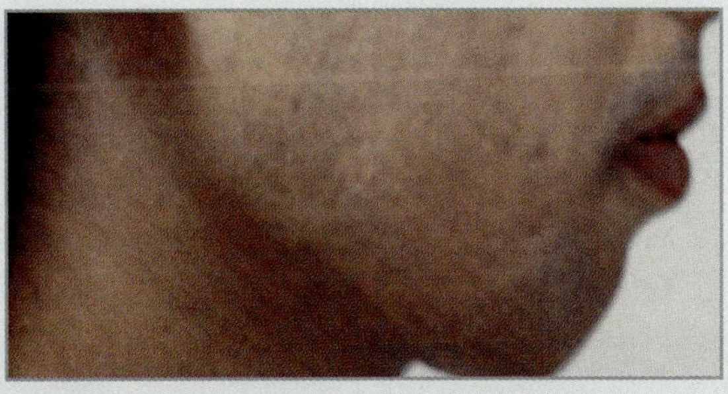

Figure 14.1: Photograph showing acne scars and severe hirsutism

INVESTIGATIONS

Complete blood count, renal, and liver functions were normal. Fasting glucose was 87 mg/dL.

- Thyroid-stimulating hormone: 2.07 mIU/mL (normal: 0.27–4.2 mIU/mL)
- Luteinizing hormone: 1.14 mIU/mL (normal: 2.4–12.6 mIU/mL)
- Follicle-stimulating hormone: 2.03 mIU/mL (normal: 3.5–12.5 mIU/mL)
- Total testosterone: 2.42 ng/mL (normal range for women 0.029–0.408 ng/mL)
- Prolactin: 15.32 ng/mL (normal: 6.0–29.9 ng/mL)
- 8AM Cortisol: 9.43 µg/dL (normal: 6.2–19.4 µg/dL)
- Adrenocorticotropic hormone (ACTH): 58.62 pg/mL (normal: 7.2–63.3 pg/mL)
- Dehydroepiandrosterone sulfate (DHEA-S) 864 mg/dL (normal: 98–340 mg/dL)
- 17-OH progesterone was >12.50 ng/mL (normal range for women in follicular phase 0.19–1.82 ng/mL)
- Following low dose dexamethasone suppression test (0.5 mg 6 hourly for 2 days), plasma testosterone was 0.4 ng/dL, and DHEA-S was 61 mg/dL
- Ultrasonography of ovaries: Unremarkable. Computed tomography (CT) of adrenals: bilateral adrenal hyperplasia (Fig. 14.2).

DISCUSSION

Several endocrine and other disorders manifest with hirsutism. Polycystic ovary syndrome (PCOS) is the most common cause for hirsutism (Table 14.1). It (hirsutism) is present in 40–90% of European and American women with

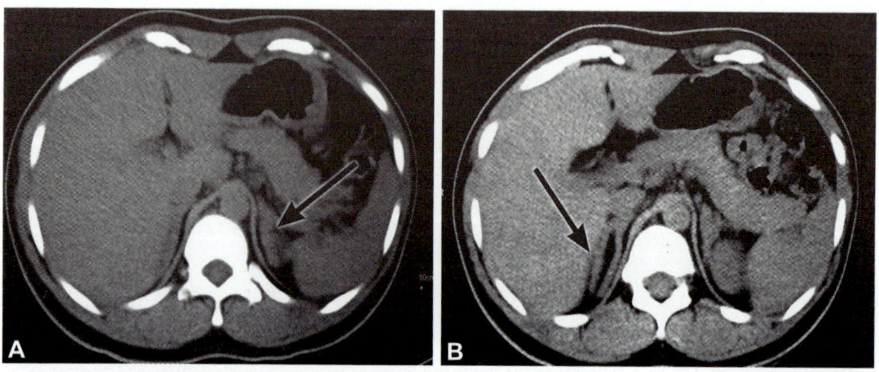

Figures 14.2A and B: **(A)** CT scan of abdomen shows the enlarged left adrenal (the arrow). **(B)** CT scan of the abdomen. The arrow points toward the right adrenal that shows diffuse hyperplasia

TABLE 14.1: Causes of hirsutism

Hirsutism with normal menses
- Ethnic variation
- Medications (minoxidil, diazoxide, cyclosporine, phenytoin, penicillamine, interferon, dexamethasone)

Hirsutism with abnormal menses
- Clinical disorders (acromegaly, Cushing's syndrome, anorexia-nervosa, porphyria cutanea tarda, hyper or hypothyroidism, acromegaly, insulin resistance, paraneoplastic syndromes)
- Medications (cyclosporine, diazoxide, minoxidil, penicillamine, dexamethasone, interferon, carbamazepine, pregablin, testosterone, antidepressants, and estrogen antagonists)
- Adrenal enzyme disorders (deficiencies)/congenital adrenal hyperplasia (CAH) (2–4%)
    - 21-hydroxylase deficiency (P450c21)
    - 11β-hydroxylase deficiency (P450c11)
    - 3β-hydroxysteroid dehydrogenase deficiency
- Neoplasms
    - Adrenal (virilizing adrenal adenoma, virilizing adrenal carcinoma) (0.2%)
    - Ovarian (Leydig cell tumor, hilus cell tumor, arrhenoblastoma)
- Persistent corpus luteum of pregnancy
- Familial ovarian hyperandrogenism
- Polycystic ovarian syndrome (PCOS) (70–80%)
- Idiopathic (4–7%)

Modified from Loriaux DL. An approach to the patient with–hirsutism. J Clin Endocrinol Metab. 2012;97:2957-68.

PCOS. It is more common among dark skinned people, rare in Japanese, and Oriental women. Several endocrine disorders like hypothyroidism, acromegaly, hyperprolactinemia, Cushing's syndrome may be associated with hirsutism. Large number of drugs (including antiepileptics and antihypertensive) can also cause hirsutism. Androgen secreting ovarian and adrenal tumors present with hirsutism and virilization. In India, we see simple virilizing forms of classical congenital adrenal hyperplasia presenting as hirsutism and primary amenorrhea during adolescence and later. Congenital adrenal hyperplasia (CAH) encompasses genetic disorders in which terminal cortisol production is impaired by mutations in genes encoding one of the enzymes or cofactors required for cortisol biosynthesis. The most common form of CAH defined often as "*classic*" CAH results from *CYP21A2* gene defect manifesting as elevated 17-hydroxyprogesterone (17-OHP), and low cortisol and aldosterone. The manifestations of 21-hydroxylase deficiency result not only from deficiencies of cortisol and aldosterone, but also from androgen excess due to shunting of accumulating precursors to 19-carbon steroids.

Diagnosis of idiopathic hirsutism is made when other causes of hirsutism are ruled out. The severity of hirsutism and the rate of progression could give some clue regarding the etiology. Ferriman–Gallwey score >16 is seen with tumoral hyperandrogenism or untreated classical congenital adrenal hyperplasia. These patients usually have primary or secondary amenorrhea. Hirsutism that appears before puberty is often caused by an ovarian or adrenal neoplasm. However, there are some benign ovarian tumors where the rate of progression may be slow and the patient may have periods. Plasma testosterone usually exceeds 2 ng/mL. Congenital hyperplasia patients rarely, if ever, have plasmas testosterone levels >2 ng/mL. Arrhenoblastoma are often large and can be detected by pelvic examination. On the other hand, lipoid cell tumors and hilus cell tumors tend to be small and may be missed on imaging.

Hirsutism is often associated with measurably elevated androgen levels, but not in all cases. Androgens in women arise from the ovary and adrenal glands, and by peripheral conversion of androgen precursors to androgens in skin and adipose tissue. A thorough history and examination are important. Laboratory investigation is essential in women with moderate to severe and/or rapidly progressing hirsutism. In mild cases identification of the underlying etiology does not alter management, but detects patients at risk for infertility, diabetes, cardiovascular disease, and endometrial carcinoma.

Our patient had long duration of symptoms, severe hirsutism, delayed menarche, irregular periods, poor breast development and signs of virilization in the form of heavy voice, marked clitoral enlargement, and some degree of posterior labial fusion. Plasma testosterone and DHEA-S were significantly increased. Elevated DHEA-S level points to hyperandrogenemia of adrenal origin. Low-dose dexamethasone suppression test revealed suppression of testosterone to normal female range. Elevated plasma, 17-hydroxy progesterone, DHEA-S also suppressed to normal female range with low-dose dexamethasone. This supported the diagnosis of congenital adrenal hyperplasia. Adrenal tumors causing hirsutism will not show consistent androgen suppression with dexamethasone. Some fluctuations in androgen levels are not uncommon in patients with tumoral hyperandrogenism as tumoral secretions can also be episodic.

The CT scan of adrenals showed hyperplasia of both adrenals in our patient.

This patient was treated with tablet dexamethasone 0.5 mg once daily, late night. A month later the dose was decreased to 0.5 mg and 0.25 mg alternate days. At this dosage, she had regular periods and breast development. Plasma testosterone reduced to low normal range. There is some appreciable difference in rate of hair growth and hair shaft diameter.

Every patient with hirsutism deserves thorough scrutiny. Once diagnosis is established, treatment depends on underlying etiology. Treatment options are drawn from menu available to clinicians that would best suit the clinical situation. Treatment strategies include cosmetic procedures (shaving, plucking, waxing); hair growth attenuation (eflornithine applied topically twice daily). It is an ornithine decarboxylase inhibitor; folliculytic therapies (lasers, electrolysis); antiandrogens (spironolactone, flutamide, finasteride, cyproterone); insulin sensitizers (includes thiazolidinediones, metformin); ovarian androgen suppression (estrogen-progestin suppression of ovarian androgen production, long-acting GnRH agonists); and disorder specific therapies such glucocorticoids for CAH. It should be noted that other than CAH, there is no indication for use of glucocorticoids in treatment of any form of hirsutism.

CONCLUSION

Hirsutism is a common clinical problem. Moderate-to-severe hirsutism and those with virilization and/or rapid progression need investigations to identify the etiology and plan specific treatment. Hirsutism with virilization, plasma testosterone >2 ng/mL or DHEA-S > 800 µg/dL are likely to be due to ovarian or adrenal tumors. In India, we do see some cases of undiagnosed/untreated classical congenital adrenal hyperplasia presenting with hirsutism. Some benign sex cord-stromal tumors of ovaries may escape detection for long periods especially in older women.

KEY POINTS

- Hirsutism is often defined in the context of cultural perceptions of normal hair distribution
- Many women who complain of hirsutism are often endocrinologically normal
- In countries where neonatal screening is not prevalent, CAH diagnosis may be delayed (particularly in nonsalt wasting type)
- Plasma testosterone exceeding 2 ng/mL or DHEA-S exceeding 800 µg/dL is highly suggestive of neoplastic process
- Some benign sex cord-stromal tumors of ovary may have long duration of symptoms. These tumors are usually small and may escape detection with imaging and even laparoscopy.

SUGGESTED READINGS

1. Auchus RJ, Arlt W. Approach to the patient: the adult with congenital adrenal hyperplasia. L Clin Endocrinol Metab. 2013;98:2645-55.
2. Goudas VT, Dumesic DA. Polycystic ovary syndrome. Endocrinol Metab Clin North Am. 1997;26(4): 893-912.
3. Somani N, Harrison S, Bergfeld WF. The clinical evaluation of hirsutism. Dermatol Ther. 2008:21(5):376-91.
4. Unluhizarci K, Kaltsas G, Kelestimur F. Non-polycystic ovary syndrome-related endocrine disorders associated with hirsutism. Eur J Clin Invest. 2012;42(1):86-94.
5. Witchel SF. Non-classic congenital adrenal hyperplasia. Curr Opin Endocrinol Diabetes Obes. 2012; 19:151-8.

CHAPTER

15

Acromegaly

Lauren A Willard, John T O'Brian

CASE PRESENTATION

Patient is a 63-year-old Caucasian female with a past medical history of hypertension, glucose intolerance, and Vitamin D deficiency, who presented originally to oral maxillary surgery section for changes in her lower jaw and ill-fitting orthodontic retainer. During the course of diagnostic evaluation that included a plain X-ray film of lateral skull, an enlarged sella was noted. The question of acromegaly was raised and referred to our endocrinology service. On laboratory evaluation, she was noted to have a markedly elevated insulin-like growth factor (IGF-1) of 1,233 ng/mL (normal for age and gender: 41–168 ng/mL) and growth hormone of 140 ng/mL (0–7.9 ng/mL).

Magnetic resonance imaging confirmed the presence of a macroadenoma with intra- and suprasellar extension, measuring 1 cm from right to left, 1.6 cm in the sagittal plane. There was evidence of left lateral displacement of pituitary gland. A note was also made of the likely invasion into the right cavernous sinus with some mass effect onto the carotid. The optic apparatus was displaced upward.

In retrospect, she endorsed enlargement of her feet and hands over a 5-year period. She reported mild weight gain over the last year. She denied having any headaches or vision changes. She had a 3-year history of hypertension. She denied arthralgia or changes in texture of skin or oily skin.

Physical examination was notable for a blood pressure of 136/82 mmHg and heart rate of 70 beats/minute on the current therapy with nonselective β/α-1 blocker. She had mild frontal bossing and prognathism. Minimal separation of her lower teeth was noted. There were sausage digits and her feet were disproportionately large. Her skin was not oily. She had an identical twin sister and the disparity in their appearance made the changes in her examination even more pronounced.

She underwent transnasal-trans-sphenoidal resection of the macroadenoma within 2 months of presentation. During her preoperative evaluation, visual field assessment was unremarkable. She also preoperatively had an echocardiogram that indicated mild left ventricular hypertrophy with preserved systolic dysfunction. Laboratories were otherwise notable for prediabetes with a glycated hemoglobin (HbA1c) of 6.3%. She had an uncomplicated postoperative course.

Immunohistochemistry of pituitary adenoma showed intense staining for human growth hormone. A few cells also showed faint staining for luteinizing hormone, but no cells stained positive for prolactin.

DIFFERENTIAL DIAGNOSIS

For this patient presenting with increasing jaw growth and sellar mass, the differential is limited. However, as our discussion outlines below, patients with acromegaly can also endorse weight gain, sweating, heat intolerance, oily skin, and acanthosis with insulin resistance, nephrolithiasis associated with hypercalciuria, fatigue, and hypogonadism. As these patients typically have a delay of diagnosis of nearly 5 years providers should be aware of more subtle presentations that may prompt testing prior to disfigurement.

MANAGEMENT

Dedicated pituitary magnetic resonance imaging (MRI) obtained 1 month after surgery indicated a small residual area of adenoma in the far right sella and repeat MRI obtained 3 months postoperatively indicated the hypoenhancing soft tissue mass in the right lateral sella appeared to be even smaller. With residual tumor she was initiated on long-acting somatostatin analog. For a short while, she was lost to follow-up.

Laboratory studies obtained approximately 16 months after adenoma resection while on continued somatostatin analog therapy with good compliance indicated normal growth hormone (GH) but IGF remained elevated at 221 ng/mL. Repeat imaging done in proximity to these laboratories indicated a slightly irregular 2 mm focus of soft tissue swelling along the floor and walls of the sella. Therapy was escalated shortly thereafter to include a dopamine agonist-cabergoline, and the dose was progressively titrated up to 1 mg twice a week. Repeat laboratories 8 weeks later showed a GH at 2.49 ng/mL and an IGF-1 that was persistently elevated at 304 ng/mL. Cabergoline therapy was again escalated to 1.5 mg twice a week with some improvement in the GH at 2 ng/mL and the IGF-1 to 234 ng/mL.

The patient was closely monitored and cabergoline continued to be increased in response to rising IGF-1 levels. Although follow-up MRI indicated a stable lesion at the floor of the sella and despite a dose of cabergoline 2 mg weekly and continued therapy with somatostatin analog, repeat levels indicated a GH 3.8 ng/mL and IGF-1 of 452 ng/mL. Based on these laboratories her medical therapy was intensified nearly 3 years after her resection to include a growth hormone receptor antagonist-pegvisomant, with a loading dose of 40 mg and then 10 mg daily.

She responded quite well to the addition of pegvisomant with her IGF-1 levels declining to 129 ng/mL and it was felt at this time that the cabergoline could be discontinued. However, her IGF-1 increased again off cabergoline to 267 ng/mL. For simplicity, her regimen of pegvisomant was increased to 20 mg daily and she was advised to stay on the same dose of somatostatin analog. Her IGF-1 improved to 70 ng/mL.

While on therapy she did have gallstones but otherwise has tolerated therapy well. Her glucose intolerance did continue to improve. As anticipated her bony changes are unchanged.

Unfortunately, approximately 6 years after surgery, she had to stop both the long-acting somatostatin analog and pegvisomant due to financial reasons, with her IGF-1 increasing in response to 494 mg/mL. She was resumed on cabergoline 5 mg weekly but could not afford this as well. Eventually, arrangements were made for monotherapy with long-acting somatostatin analog. Her most recent MRI showed stable changes over the last year with a very small hypoenhancing nodule of the sella on the right, which may be residual small focus of recurrent tumor. She was reassessed by neurosurgery and not felt to be a surgical candidate. She has been referred to radiation oncology due to need for ongoing medical therapy and persistent, yet stable, unresectable tumor.

DISCUSSION

Acromegaly is almost always as result of a benign somatotroph adenoma. Its name is derived from Greek with *akros* meaning extreme/extremity and *megal* meaning large. Even though it is rare, it carries with it significant economic burden due to its multisystem comorbidities and requirement for lifelong monitoring. The prevalence is estimated to be about 40–60 cases /million. Growth hormone's primary role is to mediate anabolic growth via the synthesis of IGF-1. Growth hormone hypersecretion leads to excess generation of IGF-1 from the liver, which mediates most of the effects of GH excess. Growth hormone secretion remains episodic but duration, number, and amplitude of episodes are all intensified, as opposed to the typical pattern of the highest pulse amplitude occurring with sleep. In acromegaly, no clear pattern is maintained.

Most tumors are >1 cm in size at the time of diagnosis, and 70% are considered macroadenomas (>10 mm). Tumors typically emanate from the lateral wings of the pituitary. It is rare for it to be part of multiple endocrine neoplasia type 1 (approximately 5% of cases are familial). Typically, these tumors are sporadic. Ectopic growth hormone releasing hormone (GHRH) and GH are rare causes of acromegaly and are not the emphasis of this discussion. If GH hypersecretion occurs prior to the fusion of the epiphyses of the long bones it leads to gigantism.

Unfortunately, the diagnosis of acromegaly is delayed in most patients, typically 5–10 years on average. Men and women are equally affected and the mean age at diagnosis is 40. In addition to the pain of disfigurement, it is a syndrome that encompasses significant morbidity and mortality.

Clinical features and presentation can include headaches and vision changes including the classic bitemporal hemianopsia that can occur with both nonsecretory and secretory pituitary adenomas. The classical presenting feature in acromegaly is the overgrowth of bone (the skull and mandible are most pronounced). Patients can have disfigurement with coarsening of facial features marked by increasing prominence of the supraorbital ridges. The nose becomes more pronounced and there can be enlargement of the mandible with anterior growth. Over time there can also be increased interdental spacing. Providers may find it constructive to look at previous photographs to appreciate the evolution in their changing appearance. Patients will note an increase in the size of their hands and feet, resulting in changed ring and shoe sizes. Hands can have spade-like fingers. Arthralgia due to bone and tissue overgrowth and eventual degenerative joint disease if left untreated can be disabling due to impaired ambulation and chronic pain. Carpel tunnel syndrome can be described in up to two thirds of patients.

Patients can also endorse increased sweating and heat intolerance as well as oily skin with sebaceous cysts. The excessive growth hormone results in organomegaly, particularly pronounced with the thyroid, and salivary glands. Patients can be frustrated with weight gain. They can develop hypogonadism over time, which can occur; as a result of deficiency of gonadotropins due to mass effect or elevated prolactin. The prolactin can be elevated not only due to stalk effect but also due to cosecretion of prolactin with GH, which can occur in 30–40% of GH producing adenomas. Cosecretion of TSH and α-subunit is also well documented in some adenomas producing growth hormone. Growth hormone secreting tumors account for 30% of familial-isolated pituitary adenomas (FIPA). Acromegalic patients display an increased proportion of 20 kDa GH isoform in circulation, whereas 22 kDa isoform is predominant in normal subjects.

Growth hormone excess can also lead to hypercalciuria and an increased risk of nephrolithiasis.

Particularly important in the preoperative assessment is a screen for sleep apnea. The sleep apnea of acromegaly can be central, obstructive, or mixed. It may be present in up to 70% of subjects. Providers should thoroughly investigate any complaints of increasing fatigue and lethargy.

Glucose intolerance is a hallmark of the disease. This effect is mediated by GH as opposed to IGF-1, which typically results in most of the clinical features of acromegaly, and can occur in 50–70% of patients. The GH stimulation that normally occurs in response to hypoglycemia is usually lost. There may be clinical findings indicative of insulin resistance including acanthosis of the axilla.

Often patients will have a diagnosis of hypertension that predates their diagnosis of acromegaly. Patients can have cardiomegaly with biventricular hypertrophy and this is important to screen for and assess, as poor cardiac function could preclude or delay potentially curative resection. Acromegalics also have an increased risk of colon polyposis; however, the evidence is still unclear as to whether this translates into higher risk of colon cancer. The polyps tend to occur in the right colon that can be associated with a higher risk of malignancy. Thyroid cancers occur with increased frequency in patients with acromegaly.

In evaluating, a patient with suspected acromegaly first a biochemical assessment is warranted. Outside of the elevations in GH and IGF-1 discussed below, other laboratory abnormalities observed in acromegaly include high postprandial glucose, hyperphosphatemia, and hypercalciuria.

INITIAL DIAGNOSTIC APPROACH

The diagnosis of acromegaly involves a coordinated assessment including a thorough history and physical. Biochemical assessment is key (Fig. 15.1), including IGF-1 measurement. IGF-1 has a longer half-life than GH and is elevated in nearly all patients with acromegaly. While its elevation alone can be diagnostic, this is not true in teenagers who can have elevated levels during growth spurts. There are basal fasting GH levels >10 ng/mL in 90% of patients. Other conditions that raise GH include acute illness, chronic renal failure, starvation, exercise, uncontrolled diabetes type-1 and estrogen therapy. None of these typically elicits an increase in IGF-1.

Growth hormone measurement is of better clinical significance in the diagnosis of acromegaly when it is obtained with glucose suppression. Just as hypoglycemia is a potent stimulus of GH secretion, hyperglycemia has the opposite effect. GH level should decline to <1 ng/mL after

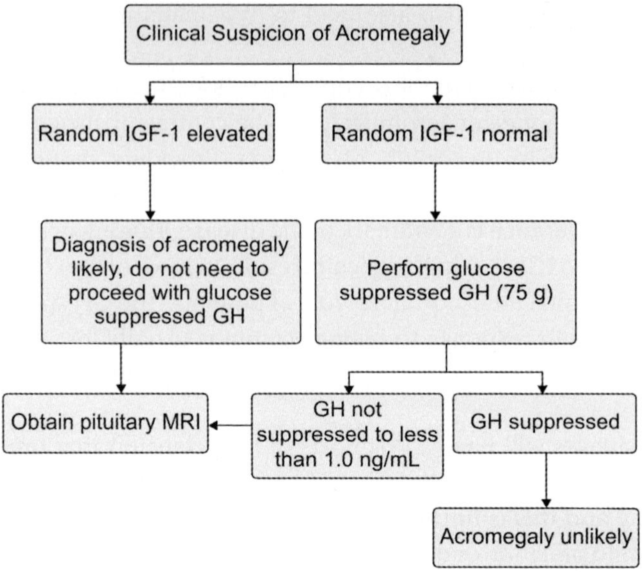

IGF-1, insulin-like growth factor; GH, growth hormone; MRI, magnetic resonance imaging.

Figure 15.1: Initial diagnostic approach

Source: Adapted from the American Association of Clinical Endocrinologist Medical Guidelines for Clinical Practice for the Diagnosis and Treatment of Acromegaly, 2011.

75–100 g of glucose. It is difficult to predict the effect the glucose will have in an acromegalic patient, but the level will not likely go below 1 ng/mL. Not used clinically now due to limited availability, recombinant thyrotropin releasing hormone (TRH) 200 μg can be administered and GH levels drawn every 20 minutes for an hour. In normal patients TRH will cause a decline in GH, acromegalic patients can have a paradoxical rise in GH. The assessment of IGF-1 and a glucose suppressed GH are crucial to biochemical assessment. Its worth pointing out that in a patient with strong suspicion for acromegaly, an oral glucose tolerance test to diagnose diabetes or glucose intolerance, an important comorbidity, can be done simultaneously with the glucose suppressed GH. Once biochemical assessment is confirmatory, a dedicated MRI of the pituitary is warranted.

Trans-sphenoidal microsurgery is the treatment of choice for intrasellar microadenomas or noninvasive macroadenomas. Patients will rarely require craniotomy if there is suprasellar extension that would not be successfully addressed with trans-sphenoidal approach. If the tumor is <2 cm, surgery is successful in treating patients in 80% of cases. Surgical complications occur in <2% of patients but enough emphasis cannot be placed on the need for an experienced neurosurgeon that performs at least 50 pituitary surgeries per year. Complications can include carotid artery injury, transient oculomotor paralysis, epistaxis, or decline in vision. Of note 40–60% of macroadenomas will not be controlled solely by surgery and will require additional medical therapy. Growth hormone immunohistochemical staining after the surgery is key to finalizing the diagnosis. Prolactin staining also has a role as there may be improved response to dopamine agonist therapy.

Somatostatin analogs also referred to as receptor ligands, act primarily at the somatostatin receptor subtypes 2 and 5 and directly inhibit GH secretion by the adenoma. It is also felt that somatostatin analogs can act indirectly to affect tumor growth by limiting angiogenesis. Initially, the formulation used was octreotide acetate, but with its inconvenient multidaily dosing regimen, it has largely been replaced by sustained release analogs such as octreotide long-acting release (LAR) and lanreotide acetate. They can shrink tumors by >20% in 75% of acromegaly patients. Typical dosing regimens of LAR consist of 20 mg monthly, increased up to 30–40 mg and then can be reduced in increments of 10 mg with good response. Lanreotide is usually started at 90 mg monthly with dose titration up to 120 mg monthly and can be reduced in increments of 60 mg. Although not frequently implemented, there is a recommendation to do a 2-week trial of short-acting somatostatin analogs before offering the long-acting formulation to assess for side effects. There is still insufficient evidence to recommend their use in the preoperative setting when surgery is planned. Patients should be counseled on possible side effects including abdominal cramping and an increased risk for gallstones and gallbladder sludge caused by reduced gallbladder contractility and altered bile composition that rarely leads to cholecystitis. Routine right upper quadrant ultrasound is not recommended unless patient becomes symptomatic. There are a few reported cases of pancreatitis as well. Typically patients need to be on therapy for 3 months before reassessing clinically and biochemically for response. Medical therapy with somatostatin analogs has been associated with improvement in headaches, fluid retention, sleep apnea, and cardiac function. Favorable response to pharmacological therapy may be predicted by tumors exhibiting low Ki index, expression of somatostatin receptor subtype 2, and wild type aryl hydrocarbon receptor interacting protein expression. Poor response would be predicted by high Ki index and presence of sparse GH tumor granulation histology.

Another option for medical therapy is dopamine agonists. Of note, while dopamine agonists typically stimulate GH secretion, they actually have a paradoxical effect in patients with acromegaly, causing a 70–80% suppression of GH. Cabergoline may be more effective than bromocriptine in this context. Cabergoline can lead to normal IGF-1 levels with only 1–2 mg/week in 30% of patients and therefore is noted to be successful as monotherapy in one third of patients. Infrequently used alone, more often cabergoline is combined with a somatostatin analog. This combination can have a 50% efficacy in reduction of GH and IGF-1 levels. There is felt to be an improved response in patients that had cosecretion of prolactin. One study demonstrated the above efficacy rates of cabergoline therapy in patients with normoprolactinemia. This raises the question as to whether cosecretion with prolactin, either noted in preoperative hyperprolactinemia or staining for prolactin on immunohistochemistry, is predictive of success with dopamine agonist therapy. Patients should be counseled on potential side effects including nausea, orthostasis, and constipation. In patients with Parkinson's disease, who are on high doses of cabergoline (typically exceeding what is used in the treatment of acromegaly) there has been an association with development of cardiac valvular abnormalities.

Pegvisomant is an engineered analog of human GH that functions as a GH receptor antagonist. It will not reduce GH secretion but acts to impair systemic effects of GH. As it does not reduce GH, its measurement can no longer be used as a marker of disease that can be followed to assess for biochemical response. The rise in endogenous GH secretion that occurs with pegvisomant occurs in a dose-dependent fashion, but typically dissipates a few weeks into therapy. Typically pegvisomant is given as a daily injection subcutaneously and has a starting dose of 10 mg and then is increased in increments of 5 mg. The average dose required is 17.4 mg. Currently, it is approved for use in patients with continued elevations of IGF-1 despite maximal therapy. In contrast to monthly injections of long-acting somatostatin analogs, pegvisomant is a daily injection, and therapy can be expensive. Tachyphylaxis has also been reported. What is promising about pegvisomant is its potential impact on the comorbidities of acromegaly. It has already been observed to significantly improve serum insulin and glucose concentrations.

Monitoring during therapy with pegvisomant should include liver function tests, particularly for elevated transaminase levels that are usually transient. Patients are often asymptomatic and the elevations and are self-limiting. These elevations can become more clinically significant in patients with diabetes and patients on combination therapy with somatostatin analogs. There is also concern that persistently elevated GH levels can result in tumor growth. A study looking at the long-term safety of pegvisomant in 1,288 subjects reported an increase in pituitary tumor size in 3.2% of the cohort.

Pasireotide is a hexapeptide that has the affinity to bind to multiple somatostatin receptors including somatostatin receptor subtypes 1, 2, 3, and 5. It has roles in other neuroendocrine tumors and Cushing's disease, but its ability to mimic endogenous somatostatin makes it a promising therapy for acromegaly as well.

Although used less frequently now, radiation therapy should be considered if the patient has poor response to surgical and medical therapy. Typical doses are 4,500–5,000 cGy. There should be consideration to the addition of somatostatin analogs in these patients as radiotherapy can take several years to have maximal effect on disease control. They will need to have withdrawal of the somatostatin analog once IGF-1 levels become normal to see if they can maintain biochemical control with just residual effects from the radiation therapy. They will continue to need to be reassessed annually for recurrence or to see if the somatostatin analog can be weaned again if previously failed.

Also of consideration is stereotactic radiosurgery including Gamma Knife, CyberKnife, linear accelerator, and proton beam. Gamma Knife has similar efficacy to standard radiation therapy. For either form of radiotherapy patients' needs to be counseled about the risk of hypopituitarism estimated to be observed in over 50% of patients. There is also concern over secondary brain tumors including *meningiomas, neuroblastoma,* and *myelogenous leukemia.* Also worth noting, particularly in patients that receive cumulative doses >50 Gy, is the risk of radiation induced optic neuropathy that can cause vision loss 10–20 months after radiation treatments. One retrospective data analysis also reported death due to cerebrovascular accident in 14.3% of patients who received conventional radiotherapy perhaps due to radiation vasculopathy.

After patients undergo surgical resection, patients should have repeat MRI at least 3 months after surgery. Edema and inflammation would have ideally resolved by this point and would not create artifact to interfere with interpretation. They will also need to have reassessment of residual pituitary function and appropriate replacement including assessment of gonadotropin function in premenopausal women.

Remission for these patients is defined as a fasting GH of <1 ng/mL or a glucose suppressed GH of <1 ng/mL as well as normal IGF-1. With more sensitive assays a GH of <0.4 ng/mL would be consistent with cure. These indices are best-reassessed 12 weeks after pituitary surgery. The definition of cure has evolved over the years, prior studies would have accepted GH values of <10 or 20 μg/L as cure; therefore, review of older literature must be done cautiously. Surgical cure rate is <50% for macroadenomas and only 25–30%

for invasive adenomas. Several characteristics have been proposed to predict poor surgical outcome: presentation of acromegaly in patients <25 years of age, extrasellar tumor growth, mixed tumors, dural invasion, cavernous sinus invasion, higher preoperative GH and IGF-1 levels, and Knosp radiological tumor grade.

In a study assessing of the quality of life and economic impact of acromegaly, it was noted that the majority of patients with acromegaly do not achieve disease control. Quality of life can be impacted long-term due to persisting cosmetic and orthopedic deformities even after treatment. With effective treatment and remission patients can have resolution or improvement in hypercalciuria, glucose intolerance, hyperhidrosis, carpel tunnel syndrome, arthralgia, photophobia, sleep apnea, hyperhidrosis, and headaches. Unfortunately, the bony changes that often lead to disfigurement do not regress.

Persistent disease after pituitary surgery can be difficult to manage. Patients who had visual field abnormalities prior to surgery or have any residual tumor in proximity to the chiasm will need reassessed by ophthalmology postoperatively. IGF-1 and GH levels are sufficient to follow for biochemical control. The GH does not need to be glucose suppressed, as this has not been found to be constructive when used outside of diagnostic evaluation. For IGF-1 there can be a wide variance in assays and it is likely constructive to try to continue to follow the same assay while monitoring the patient long term once the diagnosis is confirmed.

If GH is still elevated >1 ng/mL after surgery consideration should be given to somatostatin analogs, if somatostatin analogs fail to lead to biochemical control then therapy should be intensified with either dopamine agonist or GH receptor antagonist. Once control is achieved providers should plan on clinically reassessing and obtaining IGF-1 and GH in q6 month intervals for 2 years and then annually. Care for these complex patients must continue to involve a multidisciplinary approach with neurosurgery, ophthalmology, and endocrinology. Patients with persistent disease should always be reassessed to see if there an identifiable target on imaging that could be surgically resected. Unfortunately, repeat surgery has not consistently been associated with high cure rates. Of note, none of the medical therapies have been well explored in pregnant patients.

The cost of ongoing medical therapy can become a barrier to care as it was for our patient. Not all insurance companies will give authorization for coverage of medications. Unfortunately, this may dictate care to reattempt more definitive therapies such as repeat surgery or radiation.

KEY POINTS

- Acromegaly is predominantly caused by a growth secreting pituitary adenoma
- Diagnosis is confirmed by elevated circulating growth hormone and IGF-1 levels
- Most GH secreting tumors are benign. An increasing percentage of GH secreting tumors is being reported in FIPA patients
- Surgery is the first line of treatment
- Persistent acromegaly after surgical resection represents complex problem that requires a multispecialty approach to optimize outcomes
- Given our understanding that persistent disease after resection can occur in a large percentage of patients and recurrence can occur in 2–3% after cure, it is certainly a problem that any endocrinologist must be capable of managing and diligently coordinating postoperative care
- Providers must aim to identify and minimize comorbidities as patients with acromegaly can have an associated mortality rate that is twice that of the general population. Biochemical control can translate into improved outcomes for both morbidity and mortality.

SUGGESTED READINGS

1. Ben-Shlomo A, Sheppart M, Stephens JM, et al. Clinical, quality of life, and economic value of acromegaly disease control. Pituitary. 2011;14:284-94.
2. Carrasco CA, Gadelha M, Manavela M, et al. Aggressive tumors and difficult choices in acromegaly. Pituitary. 2014;17:S24-S29.
3. Grasso LFS, Pivonello R, Colao A. Somatostatin analogs as first line treatment in acromegaly: When is it appropriate? Curr Opin Endocrinol Diabetes Obes. 2012;19(4):288-94.
4. Guinto G, Abdo M, Zepada E, et al. Acromegaly: role of surgery in the therapeutic armamentarium. Intl J Endocrinol. 2012.
5. Katznelson L, Atkinson J, Cook DM, et al. American Association of Clinical Endocrinologist Medical Guidelines for Clinical Practice for the Diagnosis and Treatment of Acromegaly—2011 Update. Endocr Pract. 2011;Suppl 4:1-44.
6. Katznelson L. Approach to the patient with persistent acromegaly after surgery. J Clin Endocrinol Metab. 2010;95(9):4114-23.
7. Sandret L, Maison P, Chanson P. Place of cabergoline in acromegaly: a meta-analysis. J Clin Endocrinol Metab. 2011;96(5):1327-35.
8. Schofl C, Franz H, Grussendorf M, et al. Long-term outcome in patients with acromegaly: analysis of 1344 patients from the German Acromegaly Register. Eur J Endocrinol. 2012;168:39-47.
9. Van der Lely A, Biller BM, Brue T, et al. Long-term Safety of Pegvisomant in Patients with Acromegaly: Comprehensive Review of 1288 subjects in ACROSTUDY. J Clin Endocrinol Metab. 2012;97(5):1589-97.

CHAPTER

16

Cushing's Disease

Smita Gupta

CASE PRESENTATION

A 54-year-old female presented with proximal muscle weakness, easy bruising, weight gain, and worsening of hypertension. She had also noticed increasing facial hair for 6 months and fat deposition in the back of her neck. A recent laboratory test had shown high fasting blood glucose. She had history for hypertension, hyperlipidemia, and osteoporosis for past 5 years. She was on bisphosphonate therapy. There was a family history of hypertension, diabetes mellitus type 2, and coronary artery disease. She never smoked and did not drink alcohol.

On examination her blood pressure was 140/90 mmHg. She was obese but she felt that her face was fuller than before. Examination revealed dorsocervical fat pad, ecchymosis on skin, and few coarse plucked hairs on her chin. She had thin legs with mild edema and was unable to stand without taking support of the chair.

DIFFERENTIAL DIAGNOSIS

- Hypothyroidism
- Obesity
- Essential hypertension
- Cushing's syndrome
- Androgen producing ovarian or adrenal tumor
- Chronic exogenous administration of glucocorticoids
- Pseudo-Cushing's state.

INVESTIGATIONS

- Complete blood count: Normal
- Potassium: 2.2–3.2 mmol/L (normal: 3.5–5.1 mmol/L)
- Fasting plasma glucose: 130 mg/dL (normal: 65–99 mg/dL)
- Thyroid-stimulating hormone: 0.49 mIU/mL (normal: 0.34–5.6 mIU/mL)
- Plasma cortisol: 52 μg/dL (random)
- 24-hour urine-free cortisol: 1,343 g/24 hour (normal: 36–137 μg/24 hour)
- 1 mg overnight dexamethasone suppression test (DST): AM plasma cortisol 37.4 μg/dL (normal: <1.8 μg/dL)
- Total plasma testosterone: 152 ng/dL (normal: 16–48 ng/dL)
- Free testosterone: 6.6 pg/mL (normal: 0.6–3.8 pg/mL)
- Androstenedione: 1.86 ng/mL (normal: 0.13–0.82 ng/mL)
- Dehydroepiandrosterone sulfate: 678 μg/dL (normal: 64–180 μg/dL)
- Adrenocorticotropic hormone (ACTH): 197 pg/mL (normal: 10–65 pg/mL).

An ACTH-dependent Cushing's syndrome was diagnosed. This could either be Cushing's disease (pituitary adenoma) or ectopic ACTH syndrome (EAS) and rarely due to ectopic corticotropin releasing hormone (CRH) secretion.

8-mg overnight DST showed cortisol levels suppressed to 9 μg/dL (>50% suppression (baseline 30 μg/dL). A pituitary etiology (Cushing's disease) was suspected.

Pituitary magnetic resonance imaging (MRI): 7 mm right-side pituitary microadenoma.

She underwent resection of pituitary tumor and her cortisol levels were low at 0.8 μg/dL and ACTH levels came down to 17 pg/mL soon after surgery. Testosterone and other androgens also normalized postoperatively. She was started on hydrocortisone that was gradually stopped after 6 months once her morning cortisol levels normalized. She remained in remission for 5 years. A progressive rise in ACTH and cortisol along with re-emergence of her symptoms was then noted and MRI showed recurrence of pituitary tumor that was treated with repeat surgery but she persisted to have hypercortisolemia. Radiation therapy was started. While awaiting response of radiotherapy, she is being treated with pasireotide and her 24-hour urine-free cortisol levels are normal on treatment.

DISCUSSION

Cushing's disease, which is a condition resulting from pathologic hypercortisolism due to oversecretion of ACTH, accounts for about 70% of cases of Cushing's syndrome.

Centripetal fat distribution, weight gain, supraclavicular fat, and dorsocervical hump are common, but are sometimes misleading with the rising prevalence of obesity. Facial plethora, easy bruising, proximal myopathy, hypertension, and violaceous striae (>1 cm), thin and friable skin (Liddle's sign) are more specific but less sensitive findings. Children may present with weight gain and decreasing growth velocity.

Neuropsychiatric symptoms seen frequently may range from anxiety to frank psychosis (steroid psychosis). Poor wound healing and impaired defense mechanism makes them more susceptible to aggressive bronchopulmonary and superficial mucocutaneous infections. Vellus hypertrichosis of the forehead and upper cheeks and hyperpigmentation of skin may be seen.

Hypercalciuria leading to increased frequency of kidney stones and bone loss particularly in the vertebral bodies can be seen. Sexual dysfunction due to suppression of gonadotrophs is another symptom. Glucose intolerance and hypertension is commonly present. Many of the above symptoms improve when hypercortisolism is treated.

Establishing the Diagnosis of Cushing's Disease

Establishing the diagnosis of Cushing's disease is challenging. One must be careful not to screen during periods of acute concurrent illness (e.g. infections or congestive heart failure).

Screening Tests

At least two first-line or screening tests should be abnormal to establish the diagnosis of Cushing's syndrome. Additional or repeat testing is recommended if tests are slightly abnormal or discordant. Morning cortisol level, not always being elevated in patients with Cushing's syndrome, is not recommended as a screening test.

The screening tests for Cushing's disease are as follows:

1. *24-hour urine-free cortisol (performed on two different occasions)*: The excess cortisol in Cushing's syndrome saturates the cortisol-binding globulin (CBG), resulting in increase in free-cortisol excretion in urine. A level 3 times the upper limit of normal is considered positive test. It is important to remember certain medications and other conditions that can cause false positive and false negative results:
    a. *False positive*: Hyperthyroidism, sleep apnea, obesity, depression, alcoholism, polycystic ovarian syndrome, familial glucocorticoid resistance, rapid clearance of dexamethasone
    b. Digoxin, carbamazepine, fenofibrate (in high pressure or high-performance liquid chromatography assays), γ-hydroxybutyric acid

c. Increased free water clearance >5 L
d. *False negative*: Renal impairment (glomerular filtration rate <60 mL/min).

2. *Dexamethasone suppression test*: The 1-mg overnight DST: 1 mg dexamethasone is administered at 11:00 PM followed by measurement of plasma cortisol between 7:00 and 8:00 AM the next day. In the standard 2 mg DST (Liddle's test), 0.5 mg of dexamethasone is given every 6 hours for 2 days (48 hours) beginning at 9:00 AM; plasma cortisol is measured at the beginning and end of the 48-hour period. A plasma cortisol concentration of <1.8 µg/dL on either test excludes Cushing's syndrome. It has a sensitivity of 95% and specificity of 80%.
   a. False positive: Depression, mood disorder, Alzheimer dementia, obsessive compulsive disorder, acute withdrawal phase of alcoholism. Old age, sleep deprivation, weight loss
   b. Carbamazepine, phenytoin, phenobarbital rifampicin (increased clearance)
   c. Mitotane, estrogen (increase CBG)
   d. False negative: Aprepitant, fosaprepitant, itraconazole, ritonavir, fluoxetine, diltiazem, cimetidine.
3. *Late night salivary cortisol*: Increased late night salivary cortisol can distinguish between Cushing's syndrome and pseudo-Cushing's state with high accuracy. It has a 92–100% sensitivity and 93–100% specificity. Normal subjects have a nadir salivary cortisol between 11 PM and 12 AM of <4 nmol/L (145 ng/dL). Salivary cortisol is in equilibrium with plasma cortisol but concentrations are much lower than those of serum cortisol. It is independent of salivary flow rate and stable at room temperature and easy to collect. It is useful in evaluating pediatric population, cyclic, or intermittent Cushing's disease. It is recommended to be done at least twice on two separate occasions. A cortisol value >2 ng/mL (5.5 nmol/L) has a 100% sensitivity and 96% specificity for Cushing's syndrome.

   False abnormal results: Blood contamination, smoking, licorice, shift workers, altered sleep cycle, depressive illness, older age, and comorbidities as diabetes and hypertension acute sickness
4. *Serum cortisol:* Midnight sleeping and awake serum cortisol may be measured, but is a bit cumbersome and requires overnight hospitalization. A value of serum cortisol of <7.5 µg/dL is considered normal. A single measurement of <1.8 µg/dL effectively rules out Cushing's syndrome.

   Screening in special situations: In cases of adrenal incidentalomas and renal failure, 1 mg overnight dexamethasone suppression test is recommended. A 24-hour urine-free cortisol is preferred in pregnancy. Salivary cortisol measurement has also been advocated.

Establishing the Cause of Cushing's Disease

Once the presence of hypercortisolism is established, the next step is to establish whether the etiology is ACTH-dependent or independent. The ACTH is best measured by immunoradiometric assays.

ACTH levels >15 pg/mL are indicative of ACTH-dependent etiology and <5 pg/mL suggest ACTH independent (adrenal etiology). An intermediate value may be seen in both Cushing's disease and primary adrenal pathology-based syndrome. It is suggested to measure ACTH at least two times.

A CRH stimulation test in cases of equivocal ACTH may be helpful as the ACTH response is blunted in adrenal Cushing and a brisk rise in ACTH is observed in pituitary-dependent Cushing's diseases.

Adrenal imaging by adrenal computed tomography scan will further delineate the underlying pathology if a primary adrenal disorder is suspected. Most common lesion is adrenal adenoma followed by bilateral adrenal hyperplasia.

Additional testing is required to differentiate between ACTH-dependent Cushing's disease and EAS.

A rapid onset and progression of symptoms of hypercortisolemia, along with weight loss, hypertension, metabolic alkalosis and marked hypokalemia especially in a smoker and male gender, make diagnosis of EAS highly likely. The hypokalemia is due to the mineralocorticoid effect exerted by high cortisol concentration when it either saturates 11β-hydroxysteroid dehydrogenase type II enzyme in the kidney or reduces its expression.

Noninvasive tests like high dose (8 mg) dexamethasone suppression test and CRH stimulation test are recommended to distinguish between Cushing's disease and EAS.

8-mg Dexamethasone Suppression Test

After 8-mg dexamethasone administration at 11 PM, a >50% reduction in morning plasma cortisol compared to basal concentration is seen in Cushing's disease and not in ectopic ACTH secretion. This test is based on the fact that ACTH secretion by pituitary adenomas is only relatively resistant to the negative feedback regulation by glucocorticoids, while ectopic ACTH tumors are completely resistant to negative feedback inhibition. The sensitivity of the 8-mg DST for Cushing's disease is 81–82% with a specificity of 67–79%.

Corticotropin Releasing Hormone Simulation Test

Corticotropin releasing hormone is administered in a dose of 1 μg/kg as intravenous bolus and ACTH and cortisol responses are measured at 30 and

60 minutes. An increase from basal ACTH or cortisol concentration favors a diagnosis of Cushing's disease, while ectopic ACTH cases do not show any response. The CRH test has a sensitivity of 70–93% and a specificity of 88–100%.

When Cushing's disease is suspected, unenhanced, and gadolinium-enhanced high-resolution pituitary MRI is the imaging of choice. In a patient with classical presentation and supporting dynamic testing, a presence of a pituitary lesion of >6 mm may provide a definitive diagnosis of Cushing's disease and does not need further evaluation.

If the MRI and other dynamic tests are inconclusive bilateral inferior petrosal sinus sampling is performed. This is particularly helpful in about 40% of cases that have a normal-appearing MRI. The inferior petrosal sinus sampling is technically demanding and requires administration of CRH to improve the diagnostic yield. Simultaneous measurements of ACTH in the inferior petrosal sinus and periphery are needed before and after the administration of CRH. Cushing's disease is diagnosed when a sinus (central) to peripheral gradient is ≥2:1 before or ≥3:1 after CRH administration.

Management of Cushing's Disease

Untreated or inadequately treated Cushing's disease has significant mortality and morbidity due to an increased cardiovascular risk, including hypertension and metabolic syndrome, infections, osteoporosis, psychiatric symptoms, and arrested growth in children.

Initial Management

Corticotroph adenomas are mostly microadenomas (average size ~6 mm), macroadenomas are less common (~6%). Trans-sphenoidal surgery for tumor resection, commonly done via transnasal route these days, is the initial preferred treatment. This leads to immediate resolution of hypercortisolemia and eventual recovery of normal adrenal function. The initial remission rate is higher for microadenomas, ranging from 65% to 90%. The recurrence rate is higher for macroadenoma. Re-exploration is recommended when there is persistence of hypercortisolemia in immediate postoperative days. Glucocorticoid replacement is required to treat hypocortisolemia following surgery till the hypothalamic-pituitary-adrenal axis recovers. There is a 10–25% risk of recurrence at 10 years, warranting lifelong follow-up.

Treatment of Persistent or Recurrent Disease

1. *Pituitary surgery*: Repeat pituitary surgery has a lower rate of success compared to the initial surgery.

2. *Radiotherapy/radiosurgery*: Conventional fractionated radiotherapy or stereotactic radiosurgery can be used in patients with recurrent or refractory disease and in those who are poor candidates for surgery. It can be used as first-line therapy in pediatric population. The effect of this therapy is delayed for at least 9–12 months with response rate of 50–60% within 3–5 years of therapy. It also might decrease the incidence of Nelson's syndrome in patients with bilateral adrenalectomy. 30–40% of patients may later develop hypopituitarism.
3. *Surgical bilateral adrenalectomy*: It results in immediate hypocortisolemia and is indicated in refractory cases or those who cannot undergo pituitary surgery and in metastatic pituitary carcinoma. However, bilateral adrenalectomy carries the risk of development of *Nelson's syndrome*—a locally aggressive corticotroph adenoma seen in up to 47%. Whether Nelson's syndrome is a consequence of loss of negative cortisol feedback or re-enactment of the original aggressive nature of corticotroph remains controversial. Use of prophylactic irradiation of the pituitary prior to bilateral adrenalectomy to prevent Nelson's syndrome remains debatable.
4. *Medical therapy*: There are three classes of agents used to decrease hypercortisolemia:
   a. *Drugs that inhibit steroidogenesis*: These agents block one or more enzymes involved in steroid biosynthesis:
      i. *Ketoconazole* is the most widely used agent. It decreases cortisol levels in 70–80% of patients by blocking several enzymes in the steroidogenic pathway and is rapid acting. Limiting side effects include reversible liver enzyme elevation. It also has drug interactions due to potent inhibition of Cytochrome P450 enzymes. Other common side effects are gastrointestinal disturbance and gynecomastia. Dose range is 600–1,600 mg/day.
      ii. *Metyrapone*: It is also effective in 75–80% of patients. It is among the most frequently used agents in pregnancy. Hypertension, hirsutism, acne, and nausea are important side effects. Dose range is 1–4.5 g/day.
      iii. *Etomidate*: It can achieve rapid resolution of hypercortisolemia and is given as a low dose IV infusion (0.03 mg/kg IV bolus followed by infusion 0.1 mg/kg/h, maximum dose 0.3 mg/kg/h). Close monitoring is needed due to the potential for excess sedation.
      iv. *Mitotane*: It has a specific adrenolytic action and has been extensively used in adrenocortical carcinoma as adjunctive as well as palliative therapy. It has delayed onset of action and its extensive distribution in the adipose tissue gives it a long half-life. Glucocorticoid supplementation is often needed

with this medication. This drug has significant neurological and gastrointestinal side effects and can cause severe hypercholesterolemia. Dose range is 0.5–8 g/day.

v. *Aminoglutethimide*: It is not available and trilostane has limited efficacy.

vi. Combination therapy with mitotane, metyrapone, and ketoconazole can be an effective alternative when surgical treatment for severe ACTH-dependent Cushing's syndrome is not feasible.

b. Cortisol/glucocorticoid receptor antagonists:

i. *Mifepristone,* a glucocorticoid and progesterone receptor antagonist is a rapidly acting, highly effective agent. It is primarily indicated for hypercortisolemia-induced hyperglycemia and for short-term use for crisis-like state in Cushing's disease, like steroid-induced psychosis. The initial dose is 200–400 mg/day and can be increased every 2–4 weeks to a maximal dose of 400–800 mg/day. Side effects include hypokalemia, worsening of hypertension, adrenal insufficiency (in the presence of high cortisol levels), and metrorrhagia and its use in pregnant women will terminate pregnancy. The high cortisol with this agent is seen as a result of loss of negative feedback leading to ACTH-dependent cortisol production, when glucocorticoid receptor is blocked. Adrenal insufficiency has to be diagnosed clinically rather than biochemically and treated with drug discontinuation and dexamethasone.

c. Tumor-directed medical therapy:

i. *Pasireotide* is a multireceptor ligand somatostatin analog with high affinity for somatostatin receptor subtype 5, which is expressed by pituitary tumors in Cushing's disease. It causes reduction in urinary-free cortisol in 76% patients during a 15-day treatment in ACTH-dependent manner with doses 600 mcg and 900 mcg twice a day. Common adverse effects include hyperglycemia (40%), diarrhea, cholelithiasis, abnormal liver function tests, sinus bradycardia, and QT prolongation.

ii. Dopamine agonists (*bromocriptine, cabergoline*) have shown remission in only a small minority of patients. However, cabergoline may have a role when surgery has been unsuccessful.

iii. Other therapies tried include retinoic acid, peroxisome proliferator-activated receptor (PPAR-γ) agonists, and cyproheptadine.

iv. *Potential novel adrenal blocking drugs*: Inhibitors of 11β-hydroxylase and 18-hydroxylase are currently under investigation.

CONCLUSION

Cushing's disease is challenging to diagnose. However, a systematic approach to testing can lead to accurate and timely diagnosis. Pituitary tumor resection remains the preferred initial treatment. Radiotherapy and medical therapy are used in recurrent or inoperable cases. Recent advances in medical therapy seem to be promising for long-term management of hypercortisolemia. Diagnosis and management involve an interdisciplinary cooperation among endocrinologist, radiologist, and neurosurgeons.

KEY POINTS

- Diagnosis of Cushing's disease can be challenging specially in obese population
- No screening test is 100% sensitive or specific and a battery of two to three screening tests should be performed to confirm the diagnosis of Cushing's disease
- In an ACTH-dependent Cushing's disease, if the MRI shows a definitive adenoma and high-dose dexamethasone test showing >50% suppression of cortisol, it is reasonable to proceed with pituitary surgery. If the MRI does not clearly show a pituitary lesion and the noninvasive tests are nonconcordant, inferior petrosal sinus sampling is recommended to distinguish between pituitary related Cushing's disease and ectopic ACTH secretion
- Trans-sphenoidal surgery by an experienced surgeon is the primary treatment of Cushing's disease associated with an ACTH-secreting pituitary tumor
- Radiotherapy and/or medical therapy are useful in patients with unsuccessful surgery, recurrence of disease, or patients who cannot undergo surgery
- Untreated Cushing's disease carries significant morbidity and mortality.

SUGGESTED READINGS

1. Biller BMK, Grossman AB, Stewart PM, et al. Treatment of adrenocorticotropin-dependent Cushing's syndrome: a consensus statement. J Clin Endocrinol Metab. 2008;93:2454-62.
2. Boscaro M, Arnaldi G. Approach to the patient with possible Cushing's syndrome. J Clin Endocrinol Metab. 2009;94:3121-31.
3. Feelders RA, Hofland LJ. Medical treatment of Cushing's disease. J Clin Endocrinol Metab. 2013;98: 425-38.
4. Newell-Price J. Diagnosis/differential diagnosis of Cushing's syndrome: review of best practice. Best Pract Res Clin Endocrinol Metab. 2009;23(Suppl 1):S5-S14.
5. Nieman LK, Biller BMK, Findling JW, et al. The diagnosis of Cushing's syndrome: An Endocrine Society Clinical Practice Guideline. J Clin Endocrinol Metab. 2008;93:1526-40.

CHAPTER

17

Secondary Amenorrhea and Hyperprolactinemia in a Young Female

Jagdeesh Ullal, Romesh Khardori

CASE PRESENTATION

A 19-year-old female presented with 6-month history of losing weight, along with cessation of menses, accompanied by episodic periodic headaches, nausea, polyuria, and incessant thirst. She had been getting increasingly weak, and with fragmentation of wake-sleep cycle. The onset was sudden and there was no previous history of any significant health concerns. Patient had attained menarche at age 13 and her menstrual periods had remained regular with a 30–32 days cycle. Patient had normal secondary sexual characteristics. She was a nonsmoker and denied any use of recreational drugs. She was competitive swimmer but maintained a healthy body weight. Her scholastic performance had been outstanding and in last 6 months she was not able to attend college. An internist evaluated her and in turn referred her to a psychiatrist for presumed depression and possible eating disorder. She was placed on several psychotropic agents to no avail. At this stage she was seen at another medical facility where a magnetic resonance imaging of head was obtained as part of work-up for headaches. Endocrine service was consulted for further evaluation and management.

INVESTIGATIONS

- Hemoglobin: 13.2 g/dL
- Hematocrit: 40
- White blood cell count: 7.2 K/mm^3
- Serum sodium: 144 mmol/L
- Serum potassium: 3.4 mmol/L
- Aspartate transaminase/alanine transaminase: 40/44 IU/L
- Serum albumin: 4.2 g/dL
- Serum creatinine: 0.8 mg/dL

- Serum prolactin: 28 ng/mL (normal: 10–19 ng/mL)
- Thyroid-stimulating hormone (TSH): 3.00 mIU/mL (normal: 0.4–4.0 mIU/mL)
- Cortisol: 2.9 μg/dL (normal: 7–19 μg/dL)
- Adrenocorticotropic hormone (ACTH): 13.3 pmol/mL (normal: 14–65 pmol/mL)
- Follicle-stimulating hormone (FSH): 3.2 IU/L
- Luteinizing hormone (LH): 2.2 IU/L
- Estradiol: 52 pg/mL
- α-fetoprotein (AFP) <1.0 ng/mL
- Serum osmolality: 299 mOsm/kg serum water
- Urine osmolality: 120 mOsm/kg (24-hour urine output; 6–8 L).

Magnetic resonance imaging of head: A 2.8 × 2.6 cm, intensely enhancing mass in the pineal region with mass effect on tectum. Also seen was an enhancing hypothalamic mass extending into right part of mesencephalon invading into dorsal part of third ventricle and compressing aqueduct of Sylvius accompanied by internal hydrocephalus. A computed tomography obtained earlier had shown similar findings with extension of the mass downward. Pituitary stalk could not be identified even tough rest of the pituitary was clearly visible.

We are dealing with a young female with secondary amenorrhea, diabetes insipidus, and elevated serum prolactin associated with mass in the suprasellar and pineal region causing internal hydrocephalus. There are signs of increased intracranial pressure.

EXAMINATION

Patient was not in any acute distress, but avoided eye contact. She was awake and preferred to remain supine. She complained of global headache with nausea and intermittent blurring of vision. She was very thirsty and drank water ad-lib. She weighed 97 lb with body mass index (BMI) at 17.74. Heart rate was 82 beats/minute with blood pressure (BP) of 96/66 mmHg (supine). We could not check upright standing BP as she was very reluctant to stand. Her skin was soft and moist. Previous medical history was remarkable for depression and asthma. Family medical history was unremarkable.

Neurological examination was remarkable for Parinaud's syndrome (upward gaze palsy, convergence retraction nystagmus, and pseudo Argyll-Robertson pupils) consistent with compression of tectal plate.

Cardiac and pulmonary system examination was unremarkable. There was no visceromegaly and bowel sounds were normal. Remainder of physical examination was unremarkable.

DIFFERENTIAL DIAGNOSIS

- Intracranial germinoma (aka dysgerminoma, extragonadal seminoma)
- Langerhans cell histiocytosis
- Granulomatous disease (sarcoidosis, Wegener's granulomatosis, histoplasmosis, tuberculosis)
- Lymphocytic hypophysitis
- Lymphoma
- Glioma
- Tanycytoma
- Metastatic disease.

HOSPITAL COURSE

Given the constellation of symptoms and physical findings, evaluation and management focused on consequences of suprahypophyseal/pineal lesions leading to internal hydrocephalus as well as hormonal derangements of hypogonadotropic hypogonadism, elevated prolactin, and hypocortisolemia. Hypocortisolemia was considered secondary to central pathology (cortrosyn stimulation test was normal). Hypogonadotropic hypogonadism was attributed to acute sickness and concurrent nutritional deprivation. Elevated prolactin was attributed to stress. A ventriculostomy was performed to provide symptomatic relief as well as obtain cerebrospinal fluid (CSF) sample for measurement of germinoma markers—α-fetoprotein and beta-human chorionic hormone (β-hCG). Tumor markers were absent in CSF. Routine chemistry of CSF yielded only mild increase in proteins.

Following the initial brain magnetic resonance imaging, she underwent total spine MRI to rule out spinal drop metastases. None was found. This is a case of bifocal intracranial germinoma without any spinal drop metastases.

Even though patient had very impressive polyuria from diabetes insipidus, she kept up with her losses by drinking large volume of fluids because of enhanced thirst. Patient underwent ventriculocisternostomy third ventricle biopsy and the tissue obtained was submitted for histopathology. Microscopic examination revealed large cells with prominent nucleoli and small lymphocytes. Tumor cells were immunopositive for placental alkaline phosphatase and CD117. Immunostaining for β-hCG, AFP, and CD30 was negative. A definitive tissue diagnosis of germinoma was made. She responded favorably to desmopressin-alleviating polyuria.

For a while, she continued to drink more fluids primarily out of habit as evident from sodium drifting downward following desmopressin therapy. She was placed on glucocorticoid replacement with instructions to review the hypothalamic–pituitary axis following completion of treatment.

Patient was recommended cranial irradiation for definitive management of germinoma (total dose 45 Gy administered in fractionated manner). At her 3-month follow-up, serum prolactin remained elevated. Patient had gained weight and her BMI was 21.03 with a BP of 123/79 mmHg (supine).

Appropriate work-up was delayed, in this patient because of most features: weight loss, headaches, nausea, polyuria, and polydipsia and amenorrhea were ascribed to depression and eating disorder. It was only when brain imaging revealed a suprasellar/pituitary region mass that investigations were back on track.

DISCUSSION

In a patient with secondary amenorrhea simultaneous measurement of estradiol and FSH and LH helps discriminate whether primary defect is gonadal (primary hypogonadism/hypergonadotropic hypogonadism or extra gonadal—secondary hypogonadism/hypogonadotropic hypogonadism). Once this distinction is made, appropriate investigations are ordered to figure out pathology that most likely explains symptoms and the signs. In this instance since patient has hypogonadotropic—hypogonadism, attention will focus on pituitary and hypothalamus. Most often pituitary is the culprit. Pituitary lesions include prolactinoma or other hyperfunctioning/hormone secreting pituitary tumors, nonfunctioning space occupying tumors, infiltrative or inflammatory disorders, and pituitary necrosis. In hypothalamic area, inflammatory/granulomatous disorders and infiltrative disorders including tumors (primary or metastatic) should be considered as well. In conditions like chronic under nutrition/anorexia nervosa, no morphologic lesions are seen and the defect is functional. Since there was a well-defined lesion identified on initial imaging MRI, biopsy was considered as the best way to establish final diagnosis. Once it was established that the lesion was indeed germinoma, radiation oncology was consulted for initiating, and outlining treatment plan. When germinoma synchronously involves pineal gland and suprasellar region, it is called bifocal germinoma.

This case was a perfect example of a tumor making its presence known through local pressure effects (Parinaud's syndrome) and disturbances of hormone secretory processes (elevated prolactin, hypogonadotropic secretory pattern, and diabetes insipidus). Urgency of treatment depends on whether there is associated or impending neurovascular compromise such as cranial neuropathy and risk of ischemic necrosis/bleeding. When diabetes insipidus is present, treatment with desmopressin is very effective. If other hormonal deficiencies exit, replacement of glucocorticoids, and thyroid hormone takes precedence over replacement of sex steroids. It is better to review state of hypothalamic-pituitary-gonadal axis recovery when patient is not acutely ill or stressed otherwise/or receiving pain medications particularly opiates. In the present case, chances of developing long-lasting/persistent hormonal deficits remain high. At doses of radiation <30 Gy, neurocognitive and emotional functioning remain preserved according to a recent study at the Children's hospital of the University of Southern California.

Radiation therapy bears strong association with risk of hypopituitarism. Growth hormone (GH) axis is the most vulnerable, and GH deficiency can occur after low dose such as 18 Gy. The percentage of people becoming GH deficient can reach 50–100% within 3–5 years in those receiving doses of 30–50 Gy. Gonadotropin deficiency is dose dependent and is seen only in those receiving radiation doses 30–50 Gy or more. In children under age 9 years, low doses of radiation may lead to precocious puberty. With higher doses of radiation, frequency of TSH, ACTH, and gonadotropin deficiency increases substantially. Therefore, it is important to monitor these patients closely to avoid adverse consequences of both under-replacements as well as over replacement of hormones.

Germ Cell Tumors

These tumors arise from residual ectoderm, mesoderm, or endoderm. World Health Organization classifies them as germinoma and nongerminomatous germ cell tumors (GCTs) that include teratoma, embryonal carcinoma, choriocarcinoma, yolk sac tumor, and the mixed GCTs. Approximately, 50–65% of germinoma occur in pineal region and 25–35% are located in suprasellar region. Pineal region tumors are 10 times more common in males. About 90% of patients are <20 years old. There is a considerable variation in geographic incidence of intracranial GSTs being five to eight times more common in Japan and Far East compared with the United States and other Western countries. There is no good explanation for this variation. Genetic basis for GCTs has been explored and some candidate genes identified as well.

There is increase in the serum and CSF tumor derived oncoproteins chiefly AFP, β-hCG, and placental alkaline phosphatase (PLA). Pure germinoma usually has absent body fluid AFP, and β-hCG, while PLA may be present. However, tumors do stain positive for one or more markers. Unlike pineal germinoma, suprasellar germinomas have no gender predilection. In younger children with elevated β-hCG, precocious puberty may be encountered.

Even though there is dissemination to adjacent brain, prognosis is good with a 5-year survival rate of 90%. Tumor cells can seed within ventricular cavity and the CSF. Drop metastases may be seen in the spinal canal.

These lesions are highly sensitive to radiation therapy. However, she remains at risk for developing anterior pituitary hormone deficiencies that are likely to be permanent, having received radiation dose in excess of 30 Gy (3,000 cGy). Weight loss itself would contribute to hypothalamic dysfunction and the consequent amenorrhea. In anorectic patients, resumption of menses occurs at a weight gain of 2.05 kg more than the weight at which menses were lost. In one study, a weight approximately 90% of standard body weight was the average weight at which menses returned.

CASE IN CONTEXT

This case is an example of young woman with secondary amenorrhea with diabetes insipidus and intracranial neoplasm. The work-up was delayed because of history of depression, and for a while her initial weight loss was presumed to be secondary to eating disorder and depression. Amenorrhea in a previously normally menstruating female is a very sensitive index of ailment (physical or psychological) and deserves full attention.

Stepwise approaches lead to identification of pathologic basis for hormonal and metabolic dysfunction. Appropriate target-based therapy was given, and appropriate hormone replacements introduced. She will require periodic evaluation to make sure she is adequately replaced. She has been told about possible chronic hormonal replacement therapy.

KEY POINTS

- Secondary amenorrhea in previously normally menstruating females should be promptly investigated. Pregnancy still remains a leading cause and must be excluded
- Diabetes insipidus implies a central pathology when it appears in older children and adults. It must be promptly investigated to avoid consequences of volume loss
- Tumors appearing in pineal gland area should be investigated for germ cell tumor, since it is the favored site and also radiation offers a definitive treatment
- It is prudent not to assume all infundibulo-hypophysis lesions as case of lymphocytic hypophysitis, since germinoma, sarcoidosis, lymphoma, and leukemic infiltrate might be overlooked otherwise
- Biopsy of the lesion is the best way to establish diagnosis provided services of skilled neurosurgeons are available
- Gratifying results including cure of underlying may be possible with appropriate treatment modality
- Pituitary functions must be monitored and treated as necessary
- Patient with excessive water intake may be able to maintain normal serum osmolality and sodium concentration despite marked polyuria. This may result in unnecessary delay in investigations.

SUGGESTD READINGS

1. Darzy KH. Radiation-induced hypopituitarism after cancer therapy: who, how and when to test. Nat Clin Pract Endocrinol Metab. 2009;5(2):88-99.
2. Deligeoroglou E, Athanasopoulos N, Tsiaris P, et al. Evaluation and management of adolescent amenorrhea. Ann NY Acad Sci. 2010;1205:23-32.
3. Ferreira L, Silveira G, Latronico A. Approach to the patient with hypogonadotropic hypogonadism. J Clin Endocrinol Metab. 2013;98:1781-8.
4. Klein DA, Poth MA. Amenorrhea: an approach to diagnosis and management. Am Fam Phys. 2013; 87(11):781-8.
5. Mufti ST, Jamal A. Primary intracranial germ cell tumors. Asian J Neurosurg. 2012;7(4):197-202.
6. WeksbergD, Shibamoto Y, Paulino AC. Bifocal intracranial germinoma: a retrospective analysis of treatment outcomes in 20 patients and review of literature. Int J Radiat Oncol Biol Phys. 2012;82(4): 1341-51.

CHAPTER

18

Diabetes Insipidus

Mandip S Rawla, Donald W Richardson, Debashish Maji

CASE PRESENTATION

Case 1

A 51-year-old female with a history of hypertension, breast cancer, and remote history of thyroid cancer was recently discovered to have a large sellar and suprasellar mass (Fig. 18.1). The patient had a history of headaches, but recently reported some associated blurriness of vision in her left eye. She was sequentially seen by ophthalmology and neurosurgery services that led to imaging [computed tomography and magnetic resonance imaging (MRI)], which showed a sellar and suprasellar mass with a bilobed appearance, measuring 3 cm in height. There was mild mass effect on the optic chiasm and the mass splayed the floor of the third ventricle deforming the hypothalamus.

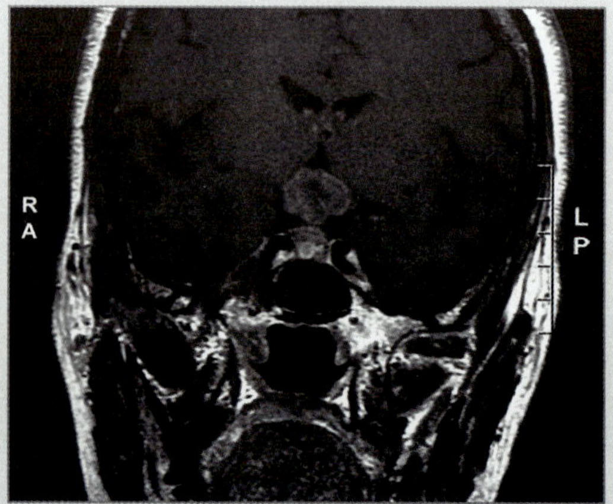

Figure 18.1: MRI pituitary showing large sellar and suprasellar mass

An endocrinology consultation was obtained prior to neurosurgery. In addition to headaches and blurry vision, her history was significant for heat and cold intolerance, sweats, and palpitations. The patient was unable to provide many details of her thyroid cancer history. It was over 20 years ago when she underwent partial resection of thyroid and adjuvant radioactive iodine treatment. She had never been on thyroid hormone replacement. In regard to her breast cancer history, she was initially diagnosed 6 years prior and underwent partial right mastectomy, chemotherapy, and radiation. Three months ago, she had an abnormal mammogram and had total mastectomy of her right breast.

Preoperative hormonal testing was performed and following results obtained:

- Thyroid-stimulating hormone: 2.39 µIU/mL (normal: 0.27–4.20 µIU/mL)
- Total T4: 3.7 µg/dL (normal: 4.5–10.9 µg/dL)
- Free T4: 0.4 ng/dL (normal: 0.9–1.8 ng/dL)
- Adrenocorticotropic hormone (ACTH): 9.2 pg/mL (normal: 7.2–63.3 pg/mL)
- Cortisol: 0.7 mg/dL (normal: 7–19 mg/dL)
- Luteinizing hormone: <0.100 mIU/mL
- Follicle-stimulating hormone: 1.4 mIU/mL
- Prolactin: 1.3 ng/mL (normal: 4.8–23.3 ng/mL).

These findings demonstrated pan-hypopituitarism. She was started on hydrocortisone 15 mg in the morning and 10 mg in the afternoon and levothyroxine 112 mg once daily. Preoperative serum sodium was 135 mmol/L (normal: 133–145), with normal renal function (serum creatinine 0.9 mg/dL).

The patient underwent right frontotemporal craniotomy and excision of the suprasellar mass. She was started on dexamethasone by neurosurgery. Intraoperatively, she made about 3 L of urine. Within 30 minutes after the surgery, the patient had an additional 925 mL of urine output. Her serum sodium increased from 143 mmol/L to 155 mmol/L. She was immediately given desmopressin 1 mg subcutaneous along with intravenous fluids. Her urine output, serum sodium, urine osmolality, and serum osmolality were followed closely. About 3 hours later, her serum sodium rose to 161 mmol/L and her urine output remained high. She was given an additional 2 mg dose of subcutaneous desmopressin with stabilization of her serum sodium and improvement in her urine osmolality from 179 to 463 mOsm/kg. Over the next 24–48 hours, the patient was able to keep up with oral hydration and intravenous fluids were discontinued. Her urine output remained high, so she was started on 200 mg desmopressin orally every night to help with nocturia. This was increased to 200 mg twice daily to control daytime urinary frequency as well. The patient remained stable on this dose with serum sodium at 138 mmol/L. In regard to her tumor, the pathology was positive for metastatic breast cancer.

Case 2

Patient is a 21-year-old Caucasian female who presented with a 3-month history of severe headaches, initially thought to represent migraines. Over time, the headaches became more severe and she underwent MRI. The MRI showed a large mass filling the frontal horns of the lateral ventricles (Fig. 18.2). Neurosurgical evaluation and biopsy showed an intraventricular grade II astrocytoma. She underwent a right frontal craniotomy and microscopic resection of

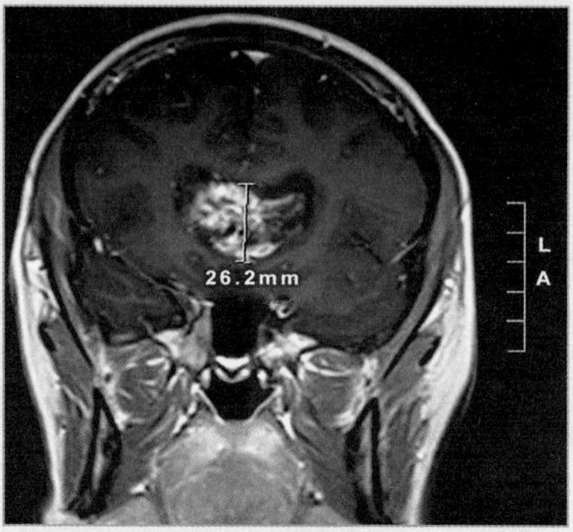

Figure 18.2: MRI brain showing a large mass filling the frontal horns of the lateral ventricles

the intraventricular tumor as well as external ventricular drain placement. Her postoperative course was significant for need for ventriculoperitoneal shunt creation and later re-exploration for proximal shunt malfunction. The patient was started on desmopressin on first postoperative day for serum sodium of 160 mmol/L with 12 L of urine output. She demonstrated cognitive impairment, including an inability to sense thirst. After 2 months postoperative recovery, she was transferred to inpatient rehabilitation. At the time of transfer, the patient was on desmopressin 1 mg subcutaneous every 12 hours. As per the records, about 24–48 hours after admission to the rehabilitation facility, the patient demonstrated tachycardia with a heart rate of 117 beats, hypotension with systolic blood pressure of 97 mmHg with the nurses noting that she was frequently incontinent of urine. Her blood chemistry revealed serum sodium of 152 mmol/L, urine osmolality of 145 mOsm/kg, and serum osmolality of 315 mOsm/kg. There were no missed doses of desmopressin but nurses noted that the patient required a lot of coaching to take her medications and would not drink any fluids. The patient was given an additional dose of IV desmopressin 1 mg and started on 0.45% normal saline intravenously. Her serum sodium, urine osmolality, and serum osmolality were monitored closely. In addition, her hypothalamic-pituitary-adrenal axis was assessed. Her 8 AM ACTH and cortisol levels were 9.3 pg/mL (normal: 7.2–63.3 pg/mL) and 10.7 µg/dL, respectively. Her free T4 was 1.6 ng/dL. Over the next several days, adjustments were made in her desmopressin dose, its route of administration, as well as her intravenous fluids. Due to her cognitive impairment, attempts to decrease her IV fluids were often unsuccessful, as the patient did not experience thirst. Nurses and family would frequently coach her to drink fluids. With desmopressin dose of 1 mg intravenous three times daily, her serum sodium was 141 mmol/L, urine osmolality was 840 mOsm/kg, and serum osmolality was 285 mOsm/kg. Her urine output was 940 mL.

As the patient was nearing transition to her next level of care in a nursing home facility, her desmopressin dose was changed to 200 µg orally twice daily. The following day, her serum sodium increased to 151 mmol/L, urine osmolality dropped to 166 mOsm/kg, and serum osmolality was 305 mOsm/kg. After several adjustments over the next few days, she stabilized on desmopressin 500 µg orally twice daily. The family was also advised that she should take in about 2 L of fluids daily. A percutaneous endoscopic gastrostomy tube to assist with administration of water was offered to the family and accepted. She now remains on desmopressin 500 µg orally twice daily and receives about 1.5 L of fluid in her feeding tube. She has not required any readmissions to the hospital since.

Case 3

A 24-year-old male presented to endocrine clinic with symptoms of increased urinary frequency, high urine volumes, and nocturia of 6 months duration. He also reported excessive daytime somnolence as a result of the nocturia as well as excessive thirst. He initially presented to his primary care physician who did an initial workup. His urine volume measured at 4.5 L in 24 hours. Further he had a normal fasting blood sugar and complete blood count. His urinalysis showed a specific gravity of 1.006. He was subsequently referred to endocrinology.

The patient denied any history of pituitary surgery, headaches, vision problems, nausea, vomiting, or change in his appetite. He was on no over the counter or prescription medications. He denied any alcohol or tobacco use. On physical examination, he appeared euvolemic and there was no cyanosis, jaundice, edema, clubbing, or any significant lymphadenopathy. His heart and lung examination did not show any abnormalities. Abdomen did not show any organomegaly.

Given his symptoms of polyuria, nocturia, and polydipsia, a provisional diagnosis of diabetes insipidus (DI) was made supported by a normal fasting blood sugar of 92 mg/dL, low urine specific gravity (1.006), and 24 hour urine output >50 mL/kg/day. At this stage, a water deprivation test was performed and results were consistent with a diagnosis of central DI.

The MRI of brain focusing on the sellar area was obtained. There was an absence of bright spot at the posterior pituitary region.

DISCUSSION

Arginine vasopressin (AVP), also known as antidiuretic hormone (ADH), is the water-retaining hormone in the body and helps to regulate osmolality. It also causes constriction of blood vessels. Vasopressin is a polypeptide hormone that is synthesized in the hypothalamus and travels down the infundibular stalk to be stored in the posterior pituitary. When vasopressin is released, it acts on the principal cells via its receptor (subtype V_2) in the collecting tubule of the kidney inducing cyclic adenosine monophosphate (cAMP) signaling cascade that then leads to translocation of AQP2 (aquaporins are a family of water channels) to apical membrane from intracellular vesicles. This results in water entering through AQP2 and traversing cytosol and exiting to the interstitium through AQP3 and AQP4. The AVP increases AQP2 protein expression through enhanced AQP2 gene transcription.

Diabetes insipidus is characterized by the excretion of large volumes of dilute urine. The term insipidus is derived from insipid that means "lack of flavor," referring to the taste of the watery urine. Patients typically present with thirst, polyuria, nocturia, and polydipsia. They may also have symptoms of an underlying neurologic disorder. Polyuria is often the main complaint and is defined as >3 L of urine output/day. This is different from patients with a urologic problem who often having frequent voiding with small quantities of urine. Further, osmotic diuresis can also present with polyuria such as during the recovery phase of acute kidney injury or with poorly controlled diabetes mellitus. These can be ruled out with simple blood tests.

The differential diagnosis of polyuria includes primary polydipsia, central DI, osmotic diuresis (diabetes mellitus), and nephrogenic diabetes insipidus (NDI).

Primary polydipsia, also known as psychogenic polydipsia, is characterized by excessive water intake. It can be induced by hypothalamic lesions that cause excessive thirst, by medications that cause dry mouth, or by psychiatric conditions. As opposed to DI, primary polydipsia is typically characterized by a normal to low-plasma sodium level along with a low urine osmolality.

Nephrogenic diabetes insipidus occurs when there is resistance to the action of ADH at the level of the kidney. This can be from congenital causes (AVP receptor mutations), medications such as lithium, hypercalcemia, severe hypokalemia, or from renal diseases such as *polycystic kidney disease* where the normal renal architecture is distorted. The most common cause of nephrogenic DI is aging. By definition, NDI is resistant to standard doses of vasopressin or its analog, desmopressin. Abnormalities of AQP2 would explain a type of autosomal recessive hereditary NDI. This would be reflected by absence of AQP2 excretion in response to vasopressin (patients with central DI have absence of AQP2 in urine, but show increased excretion in response to vasopressin administration). However, AQP2 assays are not readily available. The X-linked form of NDI secondary to mutations in the gene encoding the vasopressin-2 receptor (V2R) is difficult to treat. Currently, available treatments do not offer cure, but only relieve symptoms to a certain extent. In most cases, the V2R mutations are missense mutations that lead to its retention in the endoplasmic reticulum (ER), but do not interfere with its intrinsic functionality. The ER retention makes the V2R unavailable for AVP binding. Functional rescue of the V2R is under intense investigation using both cell permeable antagonists as well as cell permeable agonists.

As in our patient cases, central DI is associated with deficient secretion of ADH. It is also referred to as neurohypophyseal or pituitary DI. Its causes include trauma, surgery, granulomatous diseases, malignancy, anoxic brain injury, and rarely familial genetic defects. In contrast to nephrogenic DI, treatment with desmopressin is effective, which eliminates the polyuria and polydipsia.

There is a third type of diabetes insipidus known as diabetes insipidus of pregnancy or gestational DI. It usually presents in the second or third trimester and is a result of accelerated metabolism of vasopressin. The placenta produces an enzyme, cysteine aminopeptidase, or vasopressinase that causes increased metabolism of vasopressin. Treatment is with desmopressin.

DIAGNOSIS

When patients present with polyuria, quantification can be done with a 24-hour urine collection or by having them keep a log of the time and volume of urine produced during the day. Initial diagnostic tests include a serum sodium, serum osmolality, urine osmolality, and urine specific gravity. As mentioned previously, a low-serum sodium level with a low urine osmolality is usually indicative of excessive water intake as with primary polydipsia.

A high-serum sodium concentration with a low urine osmolality typically points toward DI. It is important to note though that patients with an intact thirst mechanism may not always have a high-serum sodium value. Typically, the water loss that occurs stimulates thirst and patients can maintain normal serum sodium concentrations. The exception to this is when patients have a central lesion or defect that affects thirst. These patients are very prone to hypernatremia as was demonstrated in our Case 2 above. This situation will be discussed further in the management section.

The dehydration or water deprivation test can be performed to confirm the diagnosis. The test is based on the principal that water deprivation should raise serum osmolality to near maximum threshold to stimulate AVP release from posterior pituitary (if intact).

At the start of the test, the patient is weighed and a serum sodium and serum osmolality is drawn. Thereafter, the patient is not allowed to drink fluids by mouth. Patient's body weight, urine volume, and osmolality of each voided specimen are recorded. This is continued until two consecutive urine osmolalities differ by <10% and/or the patient has lost 2% of body weight. When this point is reached, the serum sodium and serum osmolality are checked (where available, plasma vasopressin levels may be drawn). The patient is then administered 2 mg of intravenous vasopressin. Over the next 2 hours, urine output and urine osmolality are recorded. Where possible (depending on easy availability of a reliable AVP assay), measurement plasma concentrations of AVP before and at the end of water deprivation (prior to administration of exogenous AVP) and its correlation with serum and urine osmolality will allow differentiation among various types of DI more reliably.

The interpretation of the test is as follows:

Normal subjects will have <5% increase in urine osmolality over next 2 hours following administration of desmopressin, whereas:

1. *Primary polydipsia*: It will have a rise in urine osmolality as a result of fluid restriction with values up to 500–700 mOsm/kg with no further change with desmopressin.
2. *Central DI*: There is no rise in urine osmolality and undetectable or low plasma vasopressin levels. After desmopressin, the urine osmolality rises at least 50% but typically up to 200–400%.
3. *Nephrogenic DI*: Urine osmolality remains low during fluid restriction and remains low after desmopressin. Plasma vasopressin level is typically often as high as 10–20 pg/mL (normal: 0–5 pg/mL).

Of note, patients with partial central DI may have some ability to concentrate urine but there is an improvement after desmopressin is given. This test is generally reserved for adults. In children, this test is often performed in a hospital and they are not allowed to lose >5% of their body weight.

An alternate, uncommonly used, test uses a hypertonic saline infusion (Hickey–Hare test). The normal response (and the response in patients with primary polydipsia) to hypertonic saline infusion is a marked reduction in urine volume, increase in urine osmolality, and rise in urine specific gravity. This is usually evident in less than half an hour after initiation of saline infusion. The idea that administration of hypertonic saline results in release of ADH can be traced back to experiments of Gilman and Goodman in 1937.

Imaging also plays a role in the diagnosis of DI. In normal T1-weighted MRI, the posterior pituitary appears as a bright spot. This represents stored hormone and is often absent in patients with central DI. In addition, tumors or mass lesions involving a large area of the hypothalamus or involve the neurohypophyseal tracts as they converge in the pituitary stalk may cause DI. Close to 85–90% of the vasopressinergic neurons must be involved to produce DI.

MANAGEMENT

The mainstay of treatment with central DI is to reduce polyuria and improve polydipsia. Patients with an intact thirst mechanism may drink enough water to maintain normal serum sodium concentrations and stave off need for active treatment. However, children with no ready access to water will always need treatment.

Desmopressin, 1-desamino-8-D-arginine vasopressin (dDAVP), is the treatment of choice. It is a synthetic analog of the natural hormone, an 11-amino-acid peptide, and has more antidiuretic effects and less pressor activity. This is due to its selective action at the V2 receptor in the principal cell of the kidney rather than the V1 receptors in the blood vessels. It is available in intravenous, subcutaneous, intranasal, sublingual, and tablet formulations.

The intravenous and subcutaneous forms are often used in more acutely ill patients. Examples would be in postneurosurgical patients or nothing by mouth patients, or patients with impaired thirst mechanism who are prone to dehydration and sodium shifts. Dosing needs to be adjusted to each individual (vide infra). Typically after an intravenous dose is given, urine output will be reduced in 1–2 hours and the duration may last between 6 and 24 hours (Fig. 18.3).

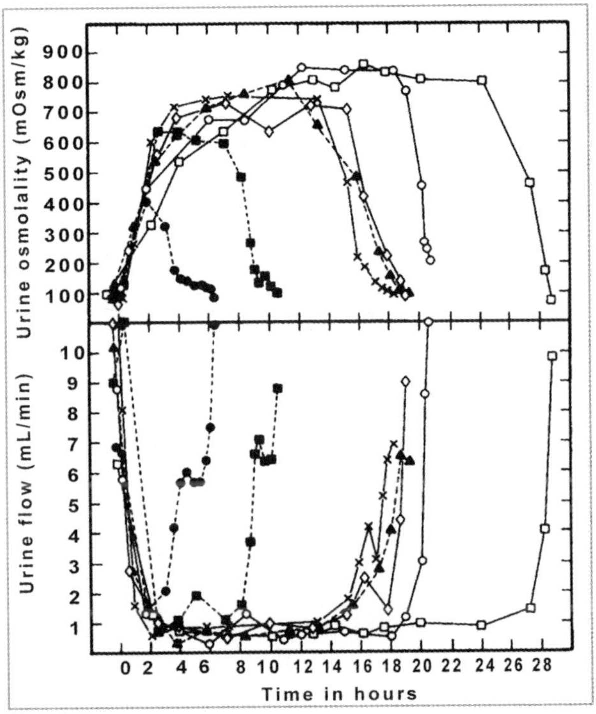

Figure 18.3: Response to intranasal and intravenous administration of desmopressin in a patient with central diabetes insipidus. Urine osmolality and flow rates are shown. Solid circles indicate intranasal doses 5 μg; solid squares indicate intranasal 10 mg; solid triangles indicate intranasal 20 μg; crosses indicate IV 1.25 μg; open diamonds indicate IV 2.5 μg; open circles indicate IV 5 μg; open squares indicate IV 10 μg.

Source: Adapted with permission from Richardson DW, Robinson AG. Drugs five years later: desmopressin. Ann Int Med. 1985;103:228-339.

Once patients are more stable, the tablet, or intranasal form may be used. The intranasal form is less bioavailable and about 5–20 times less potent than the intravenous and subcutaneous forms. The tablet form is often more preferred by patients. It comes as a 0.1 mg and 0.2 mg tablet. It typically enters the plasma about 15–30 minutes after it is taken and reaches peak concentration at about 90 minutes. Bioavailability is even less with the oral preparation, which being a peptide hormone and is variably digested before absorption. In a study using 200 or 400 μg tablets, absorption was highly variable and ranged from 0.08 to 0.16%, with up to five times higher peak concentrations after the 400 μg dose. Thus, the dose of desmopressin given orally must be determined on an individual basis and adjusted according to the response. Doses ranging from 100 to 1,200 μg given up to three times daily may be given to obtain adequate antidiuresis. Since in healthy ambulatory adults, DI is a disease and inconvenience, the authors' preference is to try once at bedtime dosing to avoid issues of positive water balance and iatrogenic syndrome of inappropriate antidiuretic hormone. This generally results in a short period of polyuria the following evening, allowing for the return of thirst and clearance of any excessive water absorption. Some patients prefer not to be bothered by polyuria at any time, in which case twice daily dosing will be needed, but a recommendation to omit one morning dose/week, presumably on a nonworking day, to allow clearance of any excess accumulation of water to occur, and prevent progressive hyponatremia.

If a patient is able to drink according to their thirst, then further dose adjustments are aimed at reducing polyuria. The patient is also instructed to drink fluids according to their thirst so as the avoid hyponatremia. Our first patient is a good example of this. Her dose was adjusted to reduce her polyuria. Again dosing is individual but strategies include giving the medication at shorter intervals such as three times daily dosing or to give the dose in the evening to reduce nocturia.

Our second patient case presents a more challenging situation. Patients with impaired thirst mechanism, infants, or disabled adults, who cannot readily acquire access to water, are more prone to dehydration and dangerous shifts in serum sodium levels. They may present with obtundation, seizures, or even coma. These patients often need intravenous fluids along with desmopressin administration. Several adjustments in the dose are often needed. If the patient is awake but unable to experience thirst, they are often prescribed a certain amount of water that they must take in throughout the day. Daily weighing by caretakers may alert the patient and medical providers to impending problems with over- or dehydration. As in our patient, the assistance of the family is often needed and may even require a feeding tube.

Third patient responded favorably to treatment with desmopressin nasal preparation (10 μg twice daily) becoming asymptomatic within 48 hours.

KEY POINTS

- Diabetes insipidus is easily diagnosed because of its abrupt onset and classic symptoms including preference for ice-cold water (pagophagia)
- Patient will present with evidence of hypertonicity (hypernatremia), polyuria and hyposthenuria (failure to concentrate urine)
- Treatment should be undertaken immediately and after completing necessary tests to determine the underlying pathology
- Medical treatment for central DI is quite effective
- Patients must be educated about proper intake of prescribed medications and avoid excessive water drinking to avoid water intoxication
- Where thirst mechanism is intact, water intake should be guided by thirst.

SUGGESTED READINGS

1. Khardori R, Ullal J, Cooperman M. Diabetes Insipidus. emedicine.medscape.com. April 10, 2014.
2. Oiso Y, Robertson GL, NØrgaard JP, et al. Treatment of neurohypophyseal diabetes insipidus. J Clin Endocrinol Metab. 2013;98(10):3958-67.
3. Richardson DW, Robinson AG. Desmopressin. Ann Int Med. 1985;103:228-339.
4. Verkman AS. Aquaporins in clinical medicine. Ann Rev Med. 2012;63:303-16.
5. Melmed S, Polonsky KS, Larsen P, et al. Williams Textbook of Endocrinology. 12th Edition. Elsevier Saunders; 2011. pg 296-304.

CHAPTER

19

Dizzy Spells in an Elderly Female

Romesh Khardori

CASE PRESENTATION

A 72-year-old female presented to urology service with complaints of urinary incontinence, recurrent abdominal pains, and dizzy spells. Her latest episode of abdominal pain had begun about 6 hours ago. Patient had normal blood counts without left shift and her renal and hepatic functions were normal. Serum electrolytes revealed hypokalemia with a serum potassium level of 3.2 mEq/L. Urinalysis was unremarkable. Patient was admitted to hospital for further evaluation and observation. Patient had history of type-2 diabetes mellitus treated with metformin 2 g daily in two divided doses and sitagliptin 100 mg once daily. Her glycated hemoglobin was 7.8%. Metformin was discontinued in anticipation of imaging studies requiring administration of contrast material, and endocrine service was consulted.

When seen by endocrine service, patient revealed long-standing history of episodic headaches associated with diaphoresis and palpitations. She further reported postural dizziness and intermittent low-grade fever. She denied history of hypertension. Physical examination revealed a heart rate (HR) of 86 beats/minute with blood pressure (BP) 146/86 mmHg in supine position. Blood pressure dropped to 96/76 mmHg in upright position, and patient felt dizzy. Her HR was 94 beats/minute. There were no other remarkable physical findings including birth marks, skin lesions, or cutaneous fibromas, or lipomas. Examination of abdomen did not reveal any palpable mass. She was placed on normal saline infusion with supplemental potassium. Two hours later patient reported chest tightness and was very diaphoretic on examination. Her HR was 88 beats/minute with a BP of 190/110 mmHg. Within 15 minutes, the BP had dropped spontaneously to 136/92 mmHg with HR of 96 beats/minute. This happened even before patient had the opportunity to take nitroglycerine for symptom of chest tightness. Patient was transferred to intensive care unit (ICU) for continuous monitoring and placement of central line. Her BP remained stable and after 12 hours of being in the ICU she underwent computed tomography scan of abdomen for persistent abdominal pain. She also demonstrated low-grade fever at 99.4°F without any evidence of infection.

DIFFERENTIAL DIAGNOSIS (POSTURAL HYPOTENSION, PAROXYSMAL HYPERTENSION, ABDOMINAL PAIN, AND FEVER)

- Pheochromocytoma (PCC)
- Diabetes mellitus type-2 with autonomic neuropathy
- Nondiabetic dysautonomia
- Porphyria
- Mesenteric angina
- Intestinal obstruction (gall stone ileus).

As part of work-up for persistent abdominal pain a computed tomography (CT) of abdomen was obtained that revealed a 3.5 × 2.4 cm cystic mass of the right adrenal gland. This was consistent with clinical suspicion of PCC. Patient was alerted to this diagnosis and further investigations were carried out at the end of the week when patient was clinically stable and without any distress.

Laboratory Data

Urine Studies

- Epinephrine: 80 μg/24 h (normal: 0–20 μg/24 h)
- Norepinephrine: 73 μg/24 h (normal: 16–80 μg/24 h)
- Metanephrine: 4,322 μg/24 h (normal: 0–1,000 μg/24 h)
- Normetanephrine: 350 μg/24 h (normal: 100–500 μg/24 h)
- Dopamine: 275 μg/24 h (normal: 65–400 μg/24 h)
- Plasma free metanephrine: 2,200 pg/mL (normal: 12–60 pg/mL)
- Plasma free normetanephrine: 76 pg/mL (normal: 0–145 pg/mL)
- Chromogranin A (CgA): 95 nmol/L (normal: 0–5 nmol/L).

DIAGNOSIS

A diagnosis of right PCC was made, and patient was prepared for surgery. She underwent right adrenalectomy without any incident and was discharged home. Histopathology confirmed a cystic tumor contained within a fibrous capsule with clear surgical margins. Nests of tumor cells demonstrated mild to moderate nuclear variability. Mitotic activity was minimal. No areas of necrosis were seen.

When seen 6 weeks late, she was asymptomatic, afebrile, and normotensive without any postural drop in blood pressure (BP). Patient had noticed improvement in blood glucose and had stopped Januvia on her own.

In retrospect, patient had long-standing symptoms but was not diagnosed sooner. Luckily, she had not sustained any end-organ damage. Had she not been in hospital where she was watched closely and investigations completed in a very short span of time, she might have had a catastrophic event when left unattended.

Final diagnosis of epinephrine secreting PCC was made. She followed up with her urologist for urinary incontinence. At the end of first year, she had remained asymptomatic with normal urinary and plasma catecholamine metabolite. Resolution of clinical and biochemical abnormalities ruled out other consideration in differential diagnosis. Incidentally but not surprisingly she had normal blood glucose with glycated hemoglobin of 5.4% despite having stopped metformin. It is inferred that patient's diabetes mellitus was instigated by PCC. Patient has remained asymptomatic, normotensive, and euglycemic at the most recent 10-year period of follow-up.

DISCUSSION

Pheochromocytomas are catecholamine secreting tumors that arise from the adrenal gland PCC or from the sympathetic ganglia [paraganglioma (PGL)] or extra-adrenal PCC. Pheochromocytoma has an estimated incidence of approximately 0.8/100,000 person years. These tumors are equally distributed across genders. Secretion of catecholamines can arise in sudden bursts giving rise paroxysmal symptoms. The classic triad of symptoms consists of palpitations, diaphoresis, and headaches lasting from few minutes to hours. Other symptoms might include panic/nervousness, nausea, blurred vision, abdominal pain, chest pain dizziness, polyuria, polydipsia, weakness, and fatigue. The typical signs include hypertension, tachycardia, orthostatic hypotension, pallor, and cardiac decompensation/cardiomyopathy. Some atypical manifestations included fever, vision impairment, constipation and intestinal obstruction (gallstone ileus), and convulsions.

Pheochromocytomas may be diagnosed under variety of scenarios:

1. Part of evaluation of resistant hypertension
2. Evaluation of patients presenting with classic symptoms
3. Incidental discovery of an adrenal mass—adrenal incidentaloma
4. Family history of PCC or familial syndromes associated with PCC [multiple endocrine neoplasia 2 (MEN2)], von Hippel-Lindau syndrome (VHL), neurofibromatosis type 1 (NF1), and familial PGL—succinate dehydrogenase (SDH)-A/AF2, B, C, D, subunit mutation].

Diagnosis of PCC rests on demonstration of unequivocal elevation of circulating catecholamines that typically include epinephrine, norepinephrine, and dopamine. Patients can present with secretion of variable amounts of each of the different catecholamines and thus present with a different clinical picture. In many patients, symptoms may be written off as nonspecific or anxiety related. Despite well-known association of hypertension, diagnosis of PCC is made in <1% of patients with hypertension.

Approximately 10–20% patient with VHL and 2% of those with NF1 develop a PCC. On the other hand, percentage of people who have PCC is much higher in MEN2 (up to 50%). Familial PGL refers to predilection in patients to develop PGLs throughout the body that may or may not produce catecholamines. This genetic syndrome is often due to a mutation in one of the SDH subunit genes. Patient with MEN2 often have higher circulating levels of epinephrine metabolite (metanephrine) compared with those with VHL and PCC, where norepinephrine metabolite (normetanephrine) might predominate. Furthermore, MEN2 patients tend to be more symptomatic and have higher incidence of paroxysmal hypertension compared with those with VHL and PCC. These patterns are not necessarily inviolable. Germ-line mutations may be seen in almost one fourth of patients with nonsyndromic PCC. Underlying germ-line mutations in 1 of 14 susceptibility genes account for 35% of PCC/PGL. For in-depth review of genetics and molecular pathogenesis of PCC and PGL reader is referred to a nice review by Galen and Kann (2013). Role of somatic or germ-line mutation in *HIF2α* gene awaits validation in larger series. Isolated cases have been reported with this mutation who presented with somatostatinomas, multiple paragangliomas, and polycythemia (*Pacak–Zhuang syndrome*).

Regarding catecholamine secretory patterns, four scenarios are possible:

1. Norepinephrine/NE-metabolite predominant
2. Epinephrine/E-metabolite predominant
3. Dopamine secreting
4. Silent/nonsecretory.

Norepinephrine dominant profile is the most common and often seen in patients with VHL mutations and extra-adrenal PCCs as well. Epinephrine dominant pattern is relatively uncommon, but may be seen in those with MEN2 or NF1 (involving *RET* and *NF1* genes respectively). Dopamine secreting PCC is uncommon. It is best diagnosed by measurement of levels of *O*-methylated metabolite of dopamine (3-methoxytyramine). Patients should be asked for any history of L-dopa prescription (such as patients with Parkinson's disease). Nonsecretory PCC is very rare.

Biochemical Testing for Diagnosis

At present measurement of plasma-free metanephrines or urinary fractionated metanephrines by mass spectrometric assays are equally recommended. A head-to-head comparison between two measurements is not available. Thus, superiority of plasma measurement versus urinary measurement remains to be established. For measurement of plasma metanephrines, blood sample should be drawn with patient in supine position for at least 30 minutes. Plasma metanephrines increase in the seated posture and thus likely to contribute to false positive results. In general, elevations of more than four times the upper limit of reference range are considered diagnostic. These tests must not be performed during any metabolic stress (trauma, infections, cerebrovascular accident). There are several medications that can interfere with measurement of metanephrines [*acetaminophen, tricyclic antidepressant (TCA), phenoxybenzamine, labetalol, sotalol, buspirone, monoamine oxidase inhibitors, cocaine, sympathomimetics, sulphasalazine,* and *levodopa*]. Interference may be analytical method specific. Labetalol and sotalol affect urinary measurements. Chromogranin A is often measured in patients with pheochromocytoma-paraganaglioma (PHEO/PGL). When combined with catecholamine measurements, the sensitivity for diagnosing PHEO/PGL comes close to 100%. The *O*-methylated metabolites (normetanephrine and metanephrine) are continuously produced due to leakage from storage vesicles of the tumor tissue and hence reflect tumor burden better than measurements of epinephrine and norepinephrine that are variable and sporadic.

If the results are equivocal, a clonidine suppression test may be in order. A glucagon stimulation test has been mentioned, but its sensitivity is too low, and it can precipitate a hypertensive crisis in those with PCC. We have used glucagon provocation test successfully in localizing PCC in a nonfamilial adult PCC presenting with bilateral adrenal nodules.

Localization

When biochemical evidence supports diagnosis of PCC/PGL, imaging is undertaken for appropriate management. In our patient, CT abdomen revealed a clear cut cystic mass. Computed tomography is preferred over magnetic resonance imaging (MRI) because of better spatial resolution. Magnetic resonance imaging is preferred in patients with metastatic disease or in those where suspicion for skull base and neck PGL is high. Magnetic resonance imaging would also be preferred in those with CT contrast allergy, whereas MRI would be contraindicated in those harboring metallic clips.

Functional imaging with metaiodobenzylguanidine (^{123}I-MIBG) is recommended when radiotherapy using ^{131}I-MIBG is planned. Accumulation of MIBG tracer may be reduced by several drugs (*sympathomimetics, cocaine, TCA, calcium channel blockers,* and *labetalol*). These drugs should be withheld for at least 2 weeks before planned study. Where ^{123}I-MIBG scanning is negative or inconclusive positron emission tomography (PET) may be helpful. A variety of radiolabelled ligands are available (^{18}F-FDG, DOPA, and ^{18}F-FDA). This technology may be expensive and not readily available in many places. Somatostatin receptor imaging has a place too because somatostatin receptors are often expressed in PCC. Receptor imaging with ^{111}In-DTA-pentetreotide (OctreoScan) is easily available in many places.

Genetic Testing

Arguments can be made for genetic testing in every patient, but certainly in those presenting before age 35 years. However, it should be done in joint consultation with the patient. Since about a quarter of patients with nonsyndromic PCC harbor germ-line mutations, establishing genetic basis in proband may prompt screening in relatives yielding earlier diagnosis. Our patient was not offered genetic testing due to nonexistent family concerns. However, a comprehensive next generation sequencing-based genetic testing strategy provides simultaneous analysis of multiple associated with predisposition to PGL and head and neck paragangliomas, thus making it a cost-effective option in investigating patients with PCC/paragangliomas. Succinate dehydrogenase mutations provide risk assessment and future prognostication very robustly.

Treatment and Management

Surgical resection is the most definitive treatment option in those diagnosed to have PCC. Most often tumor is removed by laparoscopy after the patient has been prepared properly by adequate plasma volume restoration and α-adrenergic blockade. In those with tachyarrhythmia, β-adrenoceptor or calcium channel blockers may be used in conjunction once α-adrenergic receptor blocking therapy has been instituted. α-Methyl paratyrosine that inhibits catecholamine synthesis has been used to expedite preparation for surgery. However, no uniform view about its use exists. It takes between 7 and 14 days to achieve reliable α-adrenergic blockade, and a BP target of <130/90 mmHg and a heart rate of 70–80 beats resting and 80–90 beats while standing should be acceptable.

CASE IN CONTEXT

1. Our case belongs to a rather unique category on nonsyndromic pure epinephrine secreting PCC. Patients with this kind of PCC can present with hypotension or even shock owing to desensitization of adrenergic receptors. Patients have been reported presenting with cyclic waves of hypotension alternating with hypertension. This is considered a special characteristic of epinephrine secreting tumor. Loss of baroreflex and possible cosecretion of certain vasodilators such as met-enkephalin, vasoactive intestinal polypeptide, calcitonin gene related peptide, dopamine, somatostatin may contribute to normotention/postural hypotension in these patients.
2. Our patient's type-2 diabetes would be truly considered secondary since patient required no further medical treatment following tumor excision, and her glycated hemoglobin normalized without even instituting any lifestyle changes.
3. Hypokalemia was corrected as well reflected reduced catecholamine surge.
4. Patient's protean manifestations of fever and polyuria disappeared after tumor excision.

Our case provides key lessons in looking for a unifying hypotheses and avoiding the pitfall of giving too many diagnoses that may be confounding, costly and subject patients to unnecessary treatment regimens and out of pocket expenses.

KEY POINTS

- Pheochromocytoma should be a clinical consideration at any stage of life. It is not necessarily diagnosed only in the young and middle aged
- Hormonal secretory pattern may help explain symptom constellation as well as clinical presentation
- Most PCCs are benign, and a significantly larger percentage is discovered incidentally
- It is important to follow recommendations for testing and storage of samples to avoid influence of posture, storage and transport on measurement of catecholamines, and their metabolites
- Genetic testing should be considered where yield is high and likely to impact treatment/surveillance in the patient or potentially encourage screening of family members
- Many metabolic derangements such as persistent dysglycemia, myocardial contractility, intermittent fever, abdominal cramps/obstruction may be completely resolved once PCC has been excised.

SUGGESTED READINGS

1. Conzo G, Pasquali D, Colantuoni, et al. Current concepts in pheochromocytoma. Intl J Surg. 2014;12:469.
2. Hodin R, et al. Diagnosis and management of pheochromocytoma. Current Problems in Surgery. 2014;51:151-87.
3. Kobal SL, Paran E, Jamali A, et al. Pheochromocytoma: cyclic attacks of hypertension with hypotension. Nat Clin Pract Cardiovascular Med. 2008;1:53.
4. Lenders JWM, Duh QY, Eisenhofer G, et al. Pheochromocytoma and Paraganglioma: An Endocrine Society Clinical Practice Guideline. J Clin Endocrinol Metab. 2014;99(6):1915-42.
5. Martucci VL, Pacak K. Pheochromocytoma and paraganglioma: diagnosis, genetics, management and treatment. Curr Problem Cancer. 2014;38:7.
6. Shuch B, Ricketts CJ, Metwalli AR, et al. The genetic basis of pheochromocytoma and paraganglioma: implications for management. Urology. 2014;83(6):1225-32.
7. Van Berkel A, Lenders JWM, Timmers HJLM. Biochemical diagnosis of phaechromocytoma and paraganglioma. Eur J Endocrinol. 2014;170:R109.

CHAPTER

20

Post-meal Leg Cramps: An Interesting Case of Hypokalemia

Romesh Khardori, Danielle OM Castillo

CASE PRESENTATION

A 43-year-old female presented with hypertension for preceding 10 years and recently discovered fasting blood glucose of 110 mg/dL. She had been on multiple antihypertensive medications for the past several years and these included lisinopril 20 mg twice daily; amlodipine 10 mg daily and KCL 20 mEq twice daily. Patient reported leg cramps following consumption of meals.

On physical examination, the patient weighed 127 lb. Her body mass index (BMI) was 24 kg/m^2. Her heart rate was 88 beats/minute with a blood pressure of 155/90 mmHg. Patient had otherwise a normal cardiac and pulmonary examination. Abdomen was scaphoid without any clinical evidence of organomegaly.

Patient denied family history of hypertension, cardiovascular events, or diabetes mellitus. She has had two episode of passing kidney stones.

Her recent blood chemistry was essentially normal with a serum sodium of 143 mEq/L, potassium concentration of 3.5 mEq/L, and calcium of 9.1 mg/dL. Her glycated hemoglobin was 6.3%. Patient denied any family history of hypertension or diabetes mellitus. When retested 1 hour after consumption of meal, serum potassium level had dropped to 2 mEq/L. This was confirmed after a second meal of the day as well. Patient was advised to take her potassium supplements right before her meals and remarkably her cramps resolved and repeat potassium levels were now between 3.5 mEq/L and 3.6 mEq/L. At this stage, the process began to determine underlying etiology of hypertension and meal provoked hypokalemia and renal calculi.

DIFFERENTIAL DIAGNOSIS

Based on hypertension, hypokalemia, and prediabetes/diabetes:

- Primary aldosteronism
- Pheochromocytoma (PCC)
- Cushing's syndrome
- Renovascular hypertension
- Low-renin hypertension treated with diuretics hydrochlorothiazide
- Tobacco chewing
- Excessive licorice intake (inhibits 11β-hydroxysteroid dehydrogenase).

DIAGNOSTIC WORKUP

Given long-standing history of long-standing hypertension, hypokalemia requiring potassium supplementation, and prediabetes; further investigations were undertaken after the patient was taken off lisinopril for 4 weeks and remained eukalemic with potassium supplement of 60 mEq daily. Following results obtained that included oral salt loading test:

- Blood:
    - Glucose (fasting): 103 mg/dL; HbA1c: 6.2%
    - Serum potassium: 3.4 mEq/L
    - Serum sodium: 143 mEq/L
    - Aldosterone: 21 ng/dL
    - Plasma renin activity (PRA): 0.4 ng/mL/h
    - Plasma cortisol: 11 μg/dL
    - 1-mg dexamethasone suppression test (DST): cortisol <1.2 μg/dL
    - Plasma-free metanephrine 20 pg/mL (normal: <62 pg/mL)
    - Aldosterone/renin ratio: 52.5
    - pH 7.445; HCO_3 29.3 mEq/L, BE 5.6 mmol/L.
- Urine:
    - Urinary aldosterone with sodium loading: 19 μg/24 h
    - Urine sodium: 236 mEq/24 h
    - Potassium: 74 mEq/24 h
    - Calcium: 400 mg/24 h.

Above results were consistent with hyperaldosteronism and mild metabolic alkalosis with hypercalciuria. Suppressed PRA, and normal plasma metanephrine, levels rule out renovascular hypertension, and PCC. Overnight dexamethasone suppression test rules out Cushing's syndrome. Licorice ingestion (11β-hydroxysteroid dehydrogenase inhibited/deficiency state) is ruled out by elevated aldosterone level.

Next, we proceed to obtain a computed tomography scan of the abdomen, which revealed a 6 mm right adrenal nodule. To confirm that the patient had a resectable lesion, adrenal venous sampling (AVS) was undertaken.

Adrenal venous sampling: There are two steps in interpreting AVS data. First both adrenal veins must be successfully cannulated. To confirm this, the gradient from adrenal vein to inferior vena cava (IVC) is helpful.

In order to avoid any impact from fluctuating adrenocorticotropic hormone (ACTH) levels, the AVS is carried under a constant ACTH infusion rate of 50 μg/h. The adrenal veins are sampled before and 30 minutes after ACTH stimulation. If cannula placement is correct the gradient of adrenal vein cortisol to IVC cortisol is >5:1 (generally it is even >10). Farther the cannula is away from adrenal vein, the IVC cortisol concentration decreases.

Second steps involves correcting for the dilution of left adrenal vein blood sample (cortisol concentration from left adrenal vein is usually lower than cortisol concentration from right adrenal vein due to diluting effluent from the inferior phrenic vein on the left). This is done by dividing aldosterone concentration by their corresponding cortisol concentration. Success of AVS is highly dependent on skill of the person performing the procedure. Few centers where the procedure is routinely performed must be chosen to undertake the procedure.

Adrenal venous sampling results

Measurement	Right adrenal vein	Inferior vena cava	Left adrenal vein
Aldosterone (ng/dL)	1600	40	800
Cortisol (μg/dL)	500	20	250

In this case, right adrenal vein cortisol to IVC cortisol gradient is 25, while it is 12.5 for left adrenal vein and IVC confirming correct placement of catheter. The aldosterone to cortisol ratio on right side is 3.2 and the ratio on left side is also 3.2, which fails to lateralize. Dividing right-adrenal aldosterone to cortisol ratio by the ratio obtained from left side yields ratio of 1.0 that is consistent with bilateral disease. Unilateral aldosterone excess is confirmed when the side with higher aldosterone to cortisol ratio is more than four times higher than the side with lower aldosterone to cortisol ratio. We chose medical therapy after discussion of results and treatment options/ outcomes with the patient.

DISCUSSION

Primary aldosteronism is a state of autonomous overproduction marked by hypertension and hypokalemia (provoked and unprovoked).

It is typically characterized by elevated secretion of aldosterone with suppressed PRA. In most cases, there may be an adrenal adenoma or adrenal hyperplasia. There are rare familial forms as well forms (FH-1, FH-2, and FH-3).

Primary aldosteronism results in hypertension due to volume expansion and sympathetic nervous system activation. Similar to those with primary hypertension, patients with primary aldosteronism rarely have edema. It is more prevalent in patients with resistant hypertension (20%). Aldosterone exerts its deleterious through sodium retention, potassium and hydrogen excretion, and inflammation/fibrosis. Sodium retention principally causes volume expansion. Cardiovascular events and disease are significantly increased in primary aldosteronism compared with essential hypertension. Stroke and myocardial infarction are increased 4.2-fold and 6.5-fold, respectively. There is 12-fold increase in atrial fibrillation. There is also myocardial fibrosis and ventricular hypertrophy. All these risks and complications justify a diligent search to identify a treatable cause for hyperaldosteronism.
Following categories of patients should be screened:

1. Patients with hypokalemia (unprovoked and provoked)
2. Patients with hypertension and adrenal incidentaloma
3. Patients with drug-resistant hypertension
4. Anyone where secondary hypertension is suspected
5. Young children with hypertension.

It must be noted that hypokalemia need not be present to make the diagnosis. Only a small percentage of people with primary aldosteronism have unprovoked hypokalemia (9–27%). Since aldosterone production is autonomous and independent of renin-angiotensin system, patients can be identified by ratio of plasma aldosterone concentration to PRA.

Patients are tested while seated and a ratio >30 constitutes a positive screen. When a screen is positive, investigate the patient for primary aldosteronism. It must be noted that uncorrected low potassium may reduce the aldosterone response and thus adversely affect aldosterone to renin ratio. Therefore, hypokalemia must be corrected. Sodium intake should be liberalized as well. However, potassium levels must be monitored during salt loading, since there is a risk for worsening of hypokalemia.

Primary aldosteronism is associated with higher risk of hypercalciuria, hypocitraturia, nephrocalcinosis, and nephrolithiasis.

Attention should be paid to medications that have the potential to interfere with aldosterone and/or renin measurement. Mineralocorticoid antagonists (spironolactone and eplerenone) and epithelial sodium channel inhibitor-amiloride increase both aldosterone and renin levels. Drugs like angiotensin converting enzyme inhibitors, angiotensin receptor-blockers, and potassium wasting diuretics reduce aldosterone levels and increase renin levels. Medications such as β-adrenergic blockers, central α2 adrenergic agonists, and nonsteroidal anti-inflammatory agents suppress renin levels. These drugs must be stopped for at least 4–6 weeks before screening. Patients can be placed on verapamil (slow release); methyldopa or α1-adrenergic blockers can be used so that there is the least risk of interference with aldosterone and renin measurements.

In primary aldosteronism, PRA is <1 ng/mL/h, and fails to increase above 2 ng/mL/h following furosemide administration, salt and water depletion, and/or 4 hours of upright posture/ambulation.

Following positive screen, one of the following four confirmatory tests may be used:

1. Saline suppression test
2. Fludrocortisone suppression test
3. Oral salt loading test
4. Captopril challenge test.

The saline suppression test is the most widely used confirmatory test in the United States. In this test, 2 L of 0.9% saline is infused over 4 hours. Plasma aldosterone >10 ng/dL at the end of infusion is diagnostic of primary aldosteronism.

In the fludrocortisone suppression test, plasma aldosterone is measured over a 4-day administration of fludrocortisone (0.1 mg every 6 hours) supplemented with sufficient oral slow release potassium (given 6–8 hourly) and NaCl (1,800 mg thrice daily) and high-salt diet. With the patient in an upright posture, failure to suppress aldosterone to <6 ng/dL by day 4 confirms diagnosis of primary aldosteronism.

In the oral salt loading test, urinary aldosterone levels are measured following oral salt loading (to achieve urine sodium excretion of 200 mmol/day). Potassium supplements must be provided to prevent hypokalemia. A 24-hour urine aldosterone concentration of >12 μg/24 h on the third day is diagnostic.

Once the diagnosis of primary aldosteronism has been established, the next task should be to determine what subtype of aldosteronism the patient has. Mostly patients fall into two common categories:

1. Aldosterone producing adenoma (APA)
2. Idiopathic hyperaldosteronism with unilateral or bilateral adrenal hyperplasia. The prevalence is roughly equal (50%) for either type.

It is important to establish whether the pathology is unilateral or bilateral. Unilateral disease offers a chance for permanent cure following unilateral laparoscopic adrenalectomy. Where the disease is bilateral, medical therapy with mineralocorticoid antagonist is indicated.

Imaging studies: Computed tomography, magnetic resonance imaging (MRI), and functional scanning (NP-59 scanning) may help assigning functional activity to anatomic structure. However, uncertainties still remain. Sensitivity of NP-59 depends on the size of the tumor. The tracer uptake is poor in adenomas <1.5 cm in diameter.

There are three interesting but relatively rare familial forms of primary aldosteronism:

1. Glucocorticoid-remediable hyperaldosteronism (GRA) also known as familial hyperaldosteronism type-1 (FH-1) and
2. Familial hyperaldosteronism type-2 (FH-2)
3. Familial hyperaldosteronism type-3 (FH-3).

Glucocorticoid-remediable hyperaldosteronism should be suspected in patients with onset of hypertension at a young age (<20 year age) and a family history of aldosteronism or family history of cardiovascular events at age <40 years. These individuals have a hybrid or chimeric gene that combines the ACTH responsive promoter sequence of 11α-hydroxylase gene with a distal coding sequence of aldosterone synthase gene. Thus, aldosterone synthase activity gets turned on under ACTH influence. Although the disorder was first recognized in 1966, the chimeric gene was first reported in 1992 only. A positive test for the "hybrid gene" is considered diagnostic. This has supplanted long DST to establish diagnosis. These patients demonstrate normalization of blood pressure (BP) with low doses of dexamethasone (0.25–0.5 mg/day). These patients can alternative also be effectively treated with mineralocorticoid receptor antagonists.

Familial hyperaldosteronism type-2 patients do not have the hybrid gene found in GRA. These patients are treated with mineralocorticoid receptor antagonist and carefully monitored to achieve BP control.

Familial type-3 (FH-3) is due to potassium inwardly rectifying channel subfamily J, member 5 (KCNJ5) potassium channel mutation. It was recognized recently (2011).

TREATMENT

In patients with APA, surgical removal is the most preferred treatment unless contraindicated for other reasons or patient refuses surgery. Surgery provides a cure in 50–60% of patients with marked improvement in BP control in the remainder of patients. After adrenalectomy, BP normalizes or markedly improves in the first 1–6 months, but in certain instances BP continues to improve over a year. Poor response to surgery is seen in older patients, patients with chronic hypertension, or those with coexisting primary hypertension.

Where surgery is not an option, treatment with mineralocorticoid receptor antagonists (spironolactone 12.5–50 mg/day, or eplerenone 25–100 mg/day) or amiloride 2.5–20 mg/day antagonizes aldosterone effects on the epithelial sodium channels located in renal cortical collecting ducts.

Treatment should be designed to address primary pathology and attention must be paid to electrolyte imbalance particular potassium.

Potassium supplementation may have to be significantly scaled back once mineralocorticoid receptor antagonists are introduced.

FOLLOW-UP

The patient did remarkably well; she is currently maintained on spironolactone 50 mg daily plus lisinopril 20 mg daily plus amlodipine 5 mg daily. Her potassium supplements have been reduced to 20 mEq daily. She has remained eukalemic with no further episodes of hypokalemia provoked by meals or otherwise. Incidentally, she has remained free from any renal stones and the 24-hour urine calcium has decreased to within permissible range.

We opted for lifestyle modification alone for her prediabetes state since protracted hypokalemia itself may induce glucose intolerant state. Indeed 4 months after lifestyle modification, her glycated hemoglobin was 5.7% with fasting plasma glucose at 97 mg/dL.

KEY POINTS

- Primary aldosteronism is not so rare an entity anymore. A high index of suspicion is a prerequisite for case finding when encountering individuals with long-standing and/or resistant hypertension
- Hypokalemia may be provoked by nontraditional stimuli and a careful search for etiology may be rewarding
- Initial screening should include plasma aldosterone to renin ratio keeping in mind that ratio could be altered by certain medications on board
- Adrenal venous sampling is the most definitive lateralizing test
- When the disease is bilateral, medical therapy is the most viable option
- Patients should also be evaluated for any hypercalciuria, since calcium loss, and hypocitraturia are relatively common
- Mild impairments of glucose tolerance should be reevaluated following durable return to eukalemic state.

SUGGESTED READINGS

1. Carey RM. Primary aldosteronism J Surg Oncol. 2012;106:575-9.
2. Choi M, Scholl YI, Yue P, et al. K+ channel mutations in adrenal aldosterone producing adenomas and hereditary hypertension. Science. 2011;331(6018):768-72.
3. Fuller PJ. Adrenal diagnostics: an endocrinologist's perspective focused on hyperaldosteronism. Clin Biochem Rev. 2013;34:111-6.
4. Gomez-Sanchez CE, Oki K. Minireview: potassium channels and aldosterone dysregulation: is primary aldosteronism a potassium channelopathy? Endocrinology. 2014;155:47-55.
5. Lifton RP, Dluhy RG, Powers M, et al. A chimaeric 11 β-hydroxylase/aldosterone synthase gene causes glucocorticoid remediable aldosteronism and human hypertension. Nature. 1992;355:262-5.
6. Shey J, Cameron MA, Sakhaee K, et al. Recurrent calcium nephrolithiasis with primary aldosteronism. Am J Kidney Dis. 2004;44(1):e7-12.

CHAPTER

21

Multiple Endocrine Neoplasia Type 1

David C Lieb

CASE PRESENTATION

AP is a 40-year-old woman who was referred to the endocrinology clinic for further evaluation of hypercalcemia in association with an elevated parathyroid hormone concentration. She explained that her father had been diagnosed with "multihormonal disorder" and that this condition was common on the paternal side of her family.

Past medical history is pertinent for esophageal reflux disease, but she is not currently taking any medications for this. She has history of lipoma removal, as well as a cholecystectomy. Menarche occurred at the age of 13 years, and she has had one pregnancy (with one living child who is 17 years old). She is a former smoker and rarely drinks alcohol. She is currently taking an oral contraceptive for birth control, but no other medications. Type-2 diabetes and depression are common on both sides of her family. She notes that her father had a history of parathyroid tumors requiring surgery and that he'd also been diagnosed with a pancreatic tumor. Three of her paternal aunts had been diagnosed with parathyroid disease and one had died of "pancreatic cancer." Her paternal grandmother may have had similar medical conditions.

AP notes feeling tired and cold all the time and has also been frustrated by her inability to lose weight. She also notes a poor memory. Thyroid testing has recently been normal. She suffers from occasional headaches and sinus disease, and has rare nocturia. She has also noted a low libido. Of note, she has not had any kidney stones, bone fractures, or constipation. She has not had any diarrhea, or any symptoms consistent with hypoglycemia. She has not noted any rashes. Her vision has been fine, and she has not had any breast tenderness or nipple discharge. She has had no changes in her ring or shoe size.

Outside records revealed that the patient's father had genetic testing showing a mutation in the multiple endocrine neoplasia type 1 (*MEN1*) gene.

DIFFERENTIAL DIAGNOSIS

Our patient presented with a history of hypercalcemia in association with a family history of multiple endocrine neoplasia type 1 (MEN1). In addition to MEN1, one must consider other parathyroid hormone-dependent causes of hypercalcemia, including familial hypocalciuric-hypercalcemia (FHH) and lithium-induced hypercalcemia. However, this patient is not taking lithium, and her 24-hour urine calcium was not low as would been seen in FHH. Parathyroid hormone-mediated hypercalcemia is also seen in patients with *MEN-2A* and tertiary *hyperparathyroidism*. None of these considerations was applicable to our patient.

PERTINENT INVESTIGATIONS

Evaluation for parathyroid tumors

- Plasma calcium: 10.6 mg/dL (normal: 8.4–10.5 mg/dL)
- Parathyroid hormone (intact): 112.3 pg/mL (normal: 15.0–65.0 pg/mL)
- Phosphorus: 2.1 mg/dL (normal: 2.4–4.7 mg/dL)
- 25-OH-vitamin D: 23.3 ng/mL (normal: 32.0–100.0 ng/mL)
- 1:25 dihydroxy vitamin D: 97 pg/mL (normal: 21–65 pg/mL)
- 24-hour urine calcium: 203 mg/24 h
- Glomerular filtration rate: >60 mL/min/1.73 m^2
- Bone density: Normal, including forearm measurement.

Evaluation for pancreatic neuroendocrine tumors (NETs)

- Gastrin: 54 pg/mL (normal: 0–115 pg/mL)
- Glucagon: 25 pg/mL (normal: ≤80 pg/mL)
- Vasoactive intestinal polypeptide (VIP): 13 pg/mL (normal: <75 pg/mL)
- Pancreatic polypeptide: 117 pg/mL (normal: <270 pg/mL)
- Chromogranin-A: 3 nmol/L (normal: 0–5 nmol/L)
- Fasting insulin: 12.0 uIU/mL (normal: 2.6–24.9 uIU/mL)
- Fasting glucose: 87 mg/dL (normal: <100 mg/dL)
- Abdominal CT: No pancreatic or other abdominal tumors seen.

Evaluation for pituitary tumors

- Prolactin: 16.5 ng/mL (normal: 4.79–23.3 ng/mL)
- Insulin-like growth factor-1 (IGF-1): 152 ng/mL (normal: 109–284 ng/mL)
- Pituitary/sellar MRI: No pituitary/sellar tumor seen

Evaluation for other endocrine tumors

- Chest CT: No chest (bronchial/thymic) tumors seen.

MANAGEMENT

Recommendations were made to the patient based on guidelines by Thakker et al. in the *Journal of Clinical Endocrinology and Metabolism* in June 2012.

Genetic testing: The patient was referred for genetic counseling followed by genetic testing that revealed a mutation in the *MEN1* gene; this mutation resulted in the premature truncation of the menin protein. Further management was recommended as per the algorithm shown in figure 21.1.

DISCUSSION

In June of 2012 clinical practice guidelines for the evaluation and management of MEN1 were published in the *Journal of Clinical Endocrinology and Metabolism* by Thakker et al. In these guidelines, MEN is defined as the "occurrence of tumors involving two or more endocrine glands in a single patient." Multiple endocrine neoplasia type 1 specifically involves tumors of the parathyroid glands, anterior pituitary gland, and endocrine pancreas. Multiple endocrine neoplasia type 1 may also be diagnosed in individuals with a single MEN1-associated tumor and a first-degree relative known to have MEN1, and in individuals with a known MEN1 genetic mutation (but without clinical findings suggestive of the disorder). Though the previously named endocrine organs are the most common sites of tumors in patients with MEN1, tumors of the adrenal cortex, bronchial and thymic carcinoid tumors have been described, as having nonendocrine tumors such as lipomas, fibromas, and meningiomas. The majority of individuals with MEN1 will present by their fifth decade of life, most with hyperparathyroidism. Up to 70% of patients will develop neuroendocrine tumors (NETs) of the pancreas, including gastrinoma (most common) and insulinoma, and 30–40% will develop anterior pituitary gland tumors.

Though the risk for death related to MEN1-associated tumors and tumor syndromes has decreased in recent decades, the majority of patients still die from MEN1-related illnesses, including NETs, thymic tumors, and less commonly adrenal tumors. Patients with MEN1 may not have similar outcomes when compared with their non-MEN1 counterparts.[1] Surgical cure may be more difficult, given the multiplicity of tumors, and there is an increased prevalence of metastatic and aggressive disease. Furthermore, tumors may not respond as well to typical pharmacologic and radiologic therapies.

The *MEN1* gene found on chromosome 11q13 encodes *menin*, a nuclear protein involved in gene transcription and cell proliferation. Specific MEN1 mutations do not appear to correlate with clinical phenotypes in contrast to the genotype-phenotype associations seen in patients with MEN2. However,

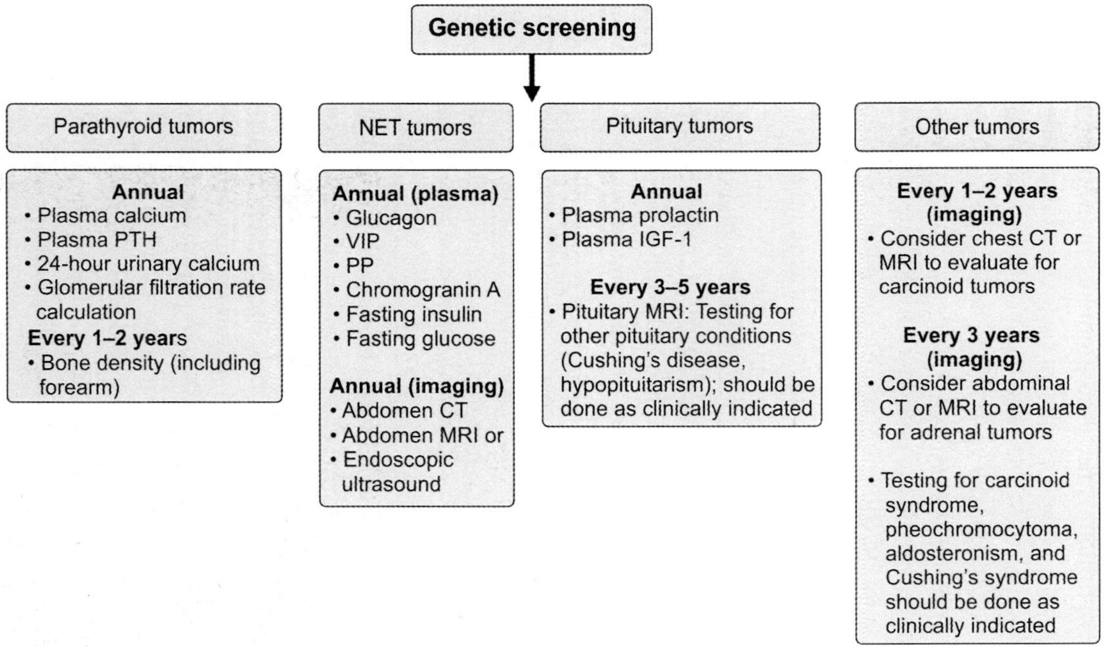

PTH, parathyroid hormone; NET, neuroendocrine tumors; CT, computed tomography; MRI, magnetic resonance imaging; VIP, vasoactive intestinal peptide; PP polypeptide, IGF-1, insulin-like growth factor 1.

Figure 21.1: Algorithm defining management strategies after a positive genetic screen

Source: Thakker et al. Algorithm summarizes recommendations described. J Clin Endocrinol Metab. 2012;97:2990-3011.

there are families of patients with MEN1 that tend to only develop parathyroid tumors (termed familial-isolated hyperparathyroidism), and these individuals may have particular missense germ-line mutations in MEN1.

All index cases of MEN1 and first-degree relatives of those with MEN1 should undergo genetic screening for mutations in the menin gene. This includes both symptomatic and asymptomatic individuals. This testing should be done as soon as there is clinical suspicion that a patient may have MEN1, as manifestations of MEN1 have been seen in patients as young as 5 years of age, and individuals <20 years of age have been described as having asymptomatic nonfunctioning pancreatic tumors. Genetic counseling should be offered to all patients given the potential consequences of positive testing. Once a mutation is found (but not before), the patient will require regular screening for the tumors and hormonal syndromes associated with MEN1.

Our patient has primary hyperparathyroidism as demonstrated by elevated calcium and parathyroid hormone (compounded by vitamin D deficiency). We, therefore, replaced her with ergocalciferol. Parathyroid disease is very common in patients with MEN1, and while patients may have similar findings and symptoms when compared with those with primary hyperparathyroidism without MEN (hypercalcemia, nephrolithiasis, musculoskeletal symptoms). However, there are significant differences. Patients may be diagnosed with hyperparathyroidism up to 30 years earlier (20s vs. 50s), with a more balanced male/female ratio. Multiple glands are typically involved in MEN1 (vs. the predominance of single parathyroid hormone adenoma in primary hyperparathyroidism), making preoperative ultrasound and sestamibi scanning somewhat less helpful. Surgical treatment options include total parathyroidectomy (removal of all four glands with autotransplantation of parathyroid tissue in the forearm) or subtotal parathyroidectomy (resection of 3.5 glands). Debate exists as to which treatment is best, as well as when to perform surgery, given the high risk for disease recurrence (up to 65% of patients undergoing subtotal parathyroidectomy). Postoperative complications include hypoparathyroidism requiring calcium and vitamin D analogs, as well as the traditional risks associated with bilateral neck surgery. The calcimimetic cinacalcet has also been used successfully to treat hyperparathyroidism in patients with MEN1. Of note, when our patient has surgery (which she most likely will at some point in the near future), we would recommend that she have a thymectomy, given the increased risk for thymic carcinoid (associated morbidity and mortality) seen in patients with MEN1.

Our patient was screened for pancreatic NETs with a variety of laboratory tests (see above). The goals of therapy in patients with NETs include reducing symptoms related to tumor bulk and hormone secretion, and to prolong life if possible. Each tumor syndrome has particular medical therapies that have been shown to reduce symptoms and possibly reduce tumor burden. There were particular concerns that she might have a gastrinoma, given its relative high incidence in patients with MEN1, and her symptoms of esophageal reflux. Gastrinoma are the most frequently encountered hormone-secreting pancreatic NETs seen in patients with MEN1 (20%, and often multiple) followed by insulinomas. Gastrinoma may metastasize to the peripancreatic lymph nodes as well as to the liver and cause the typical signs and symptoms associated with Zollinger–Ellison syndrome (ZES; peptic ulcers, diarrhea, fatty stools, associated with an increased fasting gastrin concentration). Zollinger–Ellison syndrome may be the presenting feature of MEN1 in a large group of patients with MEN1, and it may be difficult to distinguish patients with MEN1 from those without MEN1. Up to 25% of patients with MEN1 and ZES do not have a known family history of MEN. Also note that ZES may precede the diagnosis of hyperparathyroidism in up to 45% of patients. A variety of imaging modalities may be used when searching for a gastrinoma, including computed tomography (CT), magnetic resonance imaging (MRI), somatostatin-receptor scintigraphy, and endoscopic ultrasound. The medical treatment of gastrinoma involves lowering acid secretion with proton pump inhibitors and the use of H_2-receptor antagonists.

Tumors secreting glucagon and vasoactive intestinal peptide are much less common. Up to 55% of patients with MEN1 may have nonfunctioning pancreatic NETs when evaluated with endoscopic ultrasound.

Insulinomas are tumors comprised of insulin-producing β cells from the pancreatic islets, and comprise 10–30% of all NETs in patients with MEN1. Insulinomas present at an earlier age in patients with MEN1 compared to those that do not have MEN1 (<40 years). Patients may present with typical symptoms of an insulinoma (hunger, sweating, and confusion) that tend to occur with fasting, though can occur at any time. These symptoms improve after eating glucose. Diagnostic testing includes hospital admission for a supervised 72-hour fast, though evidence suggests that the majority of patients will develop symptoms within 48 hours. Endoscopic pancreatic ultrasound may be the best test for localizing an insulinoma, though CT and MRI are often utilized as well. Though agents including somatostatin analogs and diazoxide are often used to manage the symptoms associated with an insulinoma, surgery is the preferred therapy.

Glucagonomas and vasoactive intestinal polypeptide (VIP)-secreting tumors are less common in patients with MEN1 (<3% of all NETs). Patients with a glucagonoma present with the '4D syndrome': *depression, diarrhea, dermatosis* (necrolytic migratory erythema), and *deep venous thrombosis*. Patients will also often have diabetes or glucose intolerance, and often have weight loss. Occasionally, however, patients with MEN1 are asymptomatic at the time of diagnosis. Surgery is the treatment of choice, though many patients may present with metastatic disease. Somatostatin and various chemotherapy agents have been helpful in treating these individuals. The VIP-secreting tumors ("VIPomas") are associated with the Verner–Morrison syndrome: watery diarrhea, hypokalemia, and achlorhydria (WADHA). These tumors are rare in MEN1 and surgery is typically the treatment of choice. However, as with glucagonomas, chemotherapy, and medications including somatostatin analogs are often utilized.

Nonfunctioning pancreatic NETs are sometimes associated with elevations in hormones such as pancreatic polypeptide, but are not associated with a clinical syndrome. Up to 55% of patients with MEN1 will have nonfunctioning pancreatic NETs when evaluated with endoscopic ultrasound. Diagnosing these tumors is very important, as malignant nonfunctioning pancreatic NETs are a common cause of death in patients with MEN1. Imaging is recommended as early as 10 years of age. Endoscopic ultrasound may be the most sensitive test for diagnosis, while somatostatin receptor scintigraphy is very good for locating metastatic disease. When and if to perform surgery for nonfunctioning pancreatic NETs is controversial. More than half of patients with nonfunctioning tumors may have malignant disease, in which case whether to do surgery is not always clear. Those with solitary or a limited number of benign tumors isolated to the pancreas may be better surgical candidates. Recent literature has suggested a role for tyrosine kinase receptor inhibitors and mammalian target of rapamycin (mTOR) inhibitors in the management of nonfunctioning tumors, and the US Food and Drug Administration has approved the use of sunitinib (a tyrosine kinase inhibitor) and everolimus (an mTOR inhibitor) for patients with advanced disease.

All patients with MEN1 should undergo a baseline MRI of the sella to evaluate for any pituitary tumors. Patients may present with symptoms including headache and changes in vision as with non-MEN1-associated pituitary tumors. Patients need to have testing to evaluate for hypersecretory syndromes, which include hyperprolactinemia (amenorrhea, breast tenderness, galactorrhea), acromegaly (changes in ring/shoe size, hyperhidrosis, carpal tunnel syndrome), and Cushing's disease (weight gain, muscle weakness, diabetes, hypertension) especially if clinical findings suggestive of those syndromes are present. Tumors are typically treated in the same manner as in patients with non-MEN1 associated tumors. Up to 40% of patients with MEN1 may have a pituitary tumor and often times these are larger (macroadenomas) and more aggressive than pituitary tumors seen in patients without MEN1. Sixty percent of MEN1-associated pituitary tumors secrete prolactin, with growth hormone-secreting tumors being the second most common (25%). ACTH-secreting tumors are less common (5%). Tumors are sometimes plurihormonal and an increased frequency of somatolactotrophinomas has been reported. Treatment for pituitary tumors in patients with MEN1 is the same as for those without it. However, as MEN1-associated pituitary tumors tend to be larger and more aggressive, traditional therapies (surgery, dopamine receptor agonists, radiotherapy) may not be as effective.

Patients with MEN1 also have an increased incidence of carcinoid tumors, as well as adrenal tumors, thyroid tumors, lipomas, angiofibromas, collagenomas, and meningiomas. Of note, our patient has a history of having had a fatty tumor removed. While generally the treatment of these tumors is not different from that in a patient without MEN1, special attention should be given to carcinoid and adrenal tumors. Thymic carcinoid tumors in patients with MEN1 are aggressive and are a leading cause of death in patients with MEN1. Patients with carcinoid tumors are often asymptomatic and biochemical abnormalities are not always seen as might be expected. Computed tomography or MRI should be performed every 1–2 years to identify bronchial and thymic carcinoid tumors. Surgery is typically the initial therapy for patients with carcinoid tumors, though chemotherapy and radiation may be necessary.

Adrenal tumors may be seen in 20–70% of patients with MEN1, and imaging with CT or MRI is recommended every 3 years. Hormone-secreting tumors are uncommon (<10%), and tend to be aldosterone or cortisol-secreting if they do occur. Adrenal carcinoma, pheochromocytoma, and androgen-secreting tumors are rare in patients with MEN1. Tumors should be evaluated as in a patient without MEN1 (aldosterone and renin measurements, overnight low-dose dexamethasone suppression testing, fractionated metanephrines), and large tumors with concerning features on imaging should be surgically removed.

KEY POINTS

- Multiple endocrine neoplasia type 1 is a rare autosomal dominant disorder associated with tumors involving at least two endocrine glands
- Most patients will present with parathyroid disease, and pancreatic NETs and pituitary tumors are also common
- Endocrine tumors in patients with MEN1 tend to be more aggressive than in patients without MEN1 necessitating early identification and appropriate therapy
- All index cases and any first-degree relative of patient with MEN1 should be offered genetic screening after appropriate genetic counseling is performed
- Patients require frequent follow-up by a multidisciplinary group of providers that may include endocrinologist, surgeons, radiologists, pathologists, radiation oncologists, and oncologists.

SUGGESTED READINGS

1. Goudet P, Murat A, Binquet C, et al. Risk factors and causes of death in MEN1 disease. A GTE (Groupe d'Etude des Tumeurs Endocrines) cohort study among 758 patients. World J Surg. 2010;34(2):249-55.
2. Machens A, Schaaf L, Karges W, et al. Age-related penetrance of endocrine tumours in multiple endocrine neoplasia type 1 (MEN1): a multicentre study of 258 gene carriers. Clin Endocrinol (Oxf). 2007;67(4):613-22.
3. Marx SJ, Wells SA Jr. Multiple endocrine neoplasia. In: Williams Textbook of Endocrinology, 11th edition; Saunders Elsevier. 2008:1705-46.
4. Newey P, Thakker R. Role of multiple endocrine neoplasia type 1 mutational analysis in clinical practice. Endocrine Practice. 2011;17(0):8-17.
5. Thakker RV, Newey PJ, Walls GV, et al. Clinical practice guidelines for multiple endocrine neoplasia type 1 (MEN1). J Clin Endocrinol Metab. 2012;97(9):2990-3011.

CHAPTER

22

Multiple Endocrine Neoplasia Type 2

Ketan G Goswami

CASE PRESENTATION

A 25-year-old female patient is admitted to the intensive care unit (ICU) with a hypertensive crisis after labor (blood pressure >190/110 mmHg). She was nauseous during labor and received metoclopramide. She was treated for mild hypertension during pregnancy with labetalol. She is currently stable on intravenous diltiazem infusion and IV hydration. She complained of pounding headaches and anxiety episodes in the past, associated, sometimes with elevated blood pressure. She did not have consistent medical care in the past due to socioeconomic constraints. Family history is positive for her father dying at a young age from stroke and "neck swelling." In the past patient has been evaluated on different occasions by psychiatrist, neurologist, and cardiologist and was treated intermittently for anxiety, migraine, and "borderline" hypertension. On physical examination, she is a tall, thinly built female with stable vitals except mild tachycardic rhythm. She has lumpy lips on oral examination and a 2 cm right thyroid nodule. Remainder of physical examination is unremarkable (no birth marks, lumps, or nodules). Heart, lung, and abdomen examination was entirely unremarkable except for mild flank tenderness. You are consulted to rule out endocrine etiology for hypertension.

DIFFERENTIAL DIAGNOSIS

In a young patient with no prior clinical diagnosis further investigation is in order. Family history of premature vascular event and suspected thyroid issue should raise possibility of hereditary syndromes. Secondary causes of hypertension include serious endocrine conditions such as hyperaldosteronism, Cushing's syndrome, pheochromocytoma, and autonomic hyperreactivity/dysautonomia.

Abrupt withdrawal of drugs use in endocrine practice such as β-blockers, clonidine, and ACE-inhibitors may be associated with hypertensive rebound.

Pheochromocytoma can be deadly if not suspected and treated appropriately. Other diagnoses that should be considered are cardiac arrhythmias, migraine, illicit drug use, hyperthyroidism, and less commonly carcinoid, mastocytosis, medullary thyroid cancer (MTC), hypoglycemia, and syndromes associated with pheochromocytoma such as multiple endocrine neoplasia type 2 (MEN2), neurofibromatosis type 1, von Hippel-Lindau syndrome and paragangliomas. Hypotension rather than hypertension is generally seen with Carcinoid or Mastocytosis. Hypertensive crisis may be seen with porphyria. In children and young adults, mercury poisoning may be associated with hypertensive crisis.

INVESTIGATIONS

Based on the presentation, check electrolytes, renal function, complete blood count (CBC), and thyroid function. Collect 24 hour urine catecholamine and metanephrines—preferably within 24–48 hours after any significant symptomatic episode. Also, draw fasting, rested blood sample for plasma-free metanephrines. Stop medicines that can interfere with the testing of adrenal medullary hormones. These drugs include dopamine agonists, clonidine, tricyclic antidepressants, monoamine oxidase (MAO) inhibitors, non-selective β-blockers, sympathomimetics, etc. Confirm biological diagnosis before radiographic imaging. Thyroid ultrasound in our patient confirmed a right 2.3 cm nodule with other subcentimeter nodules. She underwent a fine needle aspiration of the dominant nodule. Cytology was consistent with MTC and biochemical work up showed significantly elevated calcitonin, plasma, and urinary catecholamines/metanephrines (>7–10 times upper limit of normal).

Her laboratory values are as follows:

- Plasma renin activity: 1.64 ng/mL/h (normal: 0.25–5.82 ng/mL/h)
- Aldosterone: 1 ng/dL (normal: 3–16 ng/dL)
- Calcitonin: 227 pg/mL (normal: ≤5 pg/mL),
- Plasma metanephrine: 465 pg/mL (normal: ≤57 pg/mL)
- Plasma normetanephrine: 3,180 pg/mL (normal: ≤148 pg/mL)
- Plasma total free metanephrine and normetanephrine: 3,645 pg/mL (normal: ≤205 pg/mL)
- 24 hour urinary metanephrines: 2,217 μg (normal: 90–315 μg/24 h)
- 24 hour urinary normetanephrine: 7,366 μg (normal: 122–676 μg/24 h)
- Plasma cortisol: 2.5 μg/dL (1 mg DST)
- Serum calcium, parathyroid hormone (PTH), and phosphorus were normal.

In view of available diagnostic data and clinical evaluation, multiple endocrine neoplasia type 2 (MEN2) was considered and RET (REarranged during Transfection) proto-oncogene testing was confirmatory with mutation identified at codon 918. Computed tomography of abdomen and pelvis identified a left adrenal mass of 2.7 cm.

MANAGEMENT

Pheochromocytoma should be treated aggressively first, before undertaking any invasive procedures. Use Phentolamine drip or sodium nitroprusside drip to manage hypertensive crisis. Oral regimen includes phenoxybenzamine 10 mg bid and titrated every 2–3 days until desired effect. Metyrosine (competitive inhibitor of tyrosine hydroxylase- the rate limiting step in catecholamine synthesis) may be used in dose of 250 mg every 6–8 hours as well, particularly when tumor mass is large. Cortical sparing adrenalectomy should be considered. Watch for adrenal insufficiency postoperatively and correct volume depletion and hypoglycemia appropriately. Total thyroidectomy with neck lymph node dissection should be done after pheochromocytoma is treated surgically. Monitor biochemical testing postoperatively but calcitonin may remain positive. If not symptomatic, may monitor if no metastatic disease identified.

Our patient was confirmed to have mutation in RET codon 918 and underwent successful left adrenalectomy and later thyroidectomy with neck lymph node dissection. Her symptoms improved and blood pressure is normal without need for antihypertensive treatment. Infant tested positive as well for the same mutation and was treated with prophylactic thyroidectomy after family counseling.

DISCUSSION

Multiple endocrine neoplasia type 2 syndrome is autosomal dominant with about 90% penetrance for MTC. MEN2 variants are as follows with characteristics (Table 22.1).

MEN2A syndrome accounts for >90% of MEN2 cases. MEN2B neoplasms are more aggressive than MEN2A and it is not associated with parathyroid tumors. The MEN2B syndrome accounts for about 5% of the cases of MEN2.

All MEN2 syndromes are caused by germ-line mutations in *RET* proto-oncogene located on chromosome 10 that encodes a tyrosine kinase receptor protein that is involved in activation of intracellular signaling pathways. RET is expressed in tissues of neural crest origin including C cells of thyroid, adrenal medulla, parasympathetic, sympathetic, enteric ganglia, and parathyroid cells derived from branchial arches.

TABLE 22.1: Variants of multiple endocrine neoplasia type 2	
MEN2A	MTC (70–80%), pheochromocytoma (30–50%), hyperparathyroidism (10–20%)
Familial MTC	MTC
MEN2A with cutaneous lichen amyloidosis	MEN2A and a pruritic cutaneous lesion located over the upper back
MEN2A or FMTC with Hirschsprung's disease	MEN2A or familial medullary thyroid cancer with Hirschsprung's disease
MEN2B	MTC, pheochromocytoma, intestinal and mucosal ganglio-neuromatosis, characteristic habitus, Marfanoid habitus

MEN2A, multiple endocrine neoplasia 2A; MTC, medullary thyroid cancer.

RET protein has three domains, which include an N-terminal extracellular domain that is receptor for an activated protein called glial cell derived neurotrophic factor (GDNF), a hydrophilic transmembrane domain, and an intracellular tyrosine kinase (TK) domain. The TK domain contains multiple tyrosine residues. Binding of GDNF family ligand (GFL) to RET triggers homodimerization of RET and a transformational change in the RET intracytoplasmic domain leading to autophosphorylation of the RET.

RET mutations in MEN2A are missense mutations and can be either intra or extra-cellular domain. These mutations involve codons 609, 611, 618, and 620 (exon 10) and 630, 634 (exon 11). The most frequent mutations are located in codon 634 occurring in >60% of all genetically identified MTC. MEN2B mutations are intracellular while MEN2A can be either. In MEN2A, mutations in related codons, causes activation of RET by dimerization while in MEN 2B, codon 918 (exon 16) mutation causes activated monomer in the absence of ligand and leads to activation of downstream signaling. Other mutation reported with MEN2B are in codons 883 (exon 15), and 804 (exon 14). Mutations in codons 883 and 918 are associated with younger age of onset for MTC and higher risk for metastases and mortality. Mutations have been reported in codons 768, 790, 791 (exon 13), 833, 891 (exon 15). Codon 918 is the highest risk codon.

Genetic screening should start with checking mutations in RET exons 10, 11, 13, 14, 15, and 16. If negative, then check other fifteen exons. Consider genetic work up for other inherited conditions causing pheochromocytoma such as von Hippel–Lindau disease (VHL), neurofibromatosis type 1 (NF-1), paragangliomas, etc. MEN2 syndromes are diagnosed with RET mutation analysis >99% of the time.

Medullary thyroid cancer in MEN2 is diagnosed by measuring plasma calcitonin levels: unstimulated or stimulated. Complete thyroidectomy is the treatment with removal of tumor burden including metastatic disease. The survival in patients with MTC is 86% at 5 years and 65% at 10 years. Poor prognostic factors include advanced age, advanced stage, prior neck surgery, and associated MEN2B. External radiation therapy shows no survival benefit but can be considered for palliation of locally recurrent tumors. Radioactive iodine is not useful in the treatment of patients with MTC. Palliative chemotherapy with therapies targeting receptor tyrosine kinases tyrosine kinase inhibitors (TKI) is being explored. The most studied TKIs are vandetanib, cabozantinib, motesanib, sorafenib, sunitinib, axitinib, and imatinib. Response rates vary and the data so far looks promising.

Pheochromocytoma must be ruled out or treated appropriately before undertaking invasive procedures including treatment for MTC.

MTC management is based on risk stratification:

- *Highest risk* (Level 1): MEN2B patients with mutations in codons 883, 918, and 922. In this group, complete thyroidectomy and neck lymph node dissection should be carried out as soon as possible. In infants, prophylactic thyroidectomy before age 6 months or within first month of life is indicated.
- *High risk* (Level 2): Patients with RET mutations in codons 609, 611, 618, 620, and 634 should undergo complete thyroidectomy before age 5 years.
- *Intermediate risk* (Level 3): Patients with RET mutations in codons 768, 790, 791, 804, and 891. In this group, thyroidectomy is advisable by age 5-10 year and some recommend monitoring pentagastrin-stimulated calcitonin levels.

CONCLUSION

MEN2 syndromes should be included in differential diagnosis of patients suspected of pheochromocytoma, especially with strong family history of such diagnosis or suspected cases. Medullary thyroid cancer can be diagnosed with calcitonin levels and FNA of the thyroid lesions. Medullary thyroid cancer can be aggressive in MEN2B especially with certain RET mutations as mentioned above. Genetic testing and counseling must be undertaken once MEN2 syndromes are confirmed. Monitor and treat patients based on risk stratification based on RET codon mutations. Hypertensive emergencies account for 25% of emergency department (ED) visits. The syndrome of hypertensive emergencies was first described by Volhard and Fahr (1914). JNC7 describes hypertensive crisis as a systolic BP (sBP) >179 mmHg or a diastolic BP (dBP) >109 mmHg with or without target organ involvement. The term MEN was introduced by Steiner et al., (1968) leading to designations MEN1 (formerly *Wermer's syndrome*) and MEN2 (formerly *Sipple's syndrome*). The MEN2 now subclassified into 2A and 2B.

KEY POINTS

- In familial cases of hypertension, MEN syndromes should be considered, and risk stratification undertaken
- Where pheochromocytoma co-exists, it should be treated first
- Screening young family members for mutations should be considered where testing is readily available
- Prophylactic thyroid surgery is curative when undertaken in young children.

SUGGESTED READINGS

1. Brandi ML, Gagel RF, Angeli A, et al. Consensus statement–Guidelines for Diagnosis and therapy of MEN Type 1 and Type2. J Clin Endocrinol Metab. 2001;86(12):5658-71.
2. Kloos RT, Eng C, Evans DB, et al. for ATA Task Force. Medullary thyroid cancer: Management Guidelines of the American Thyroid Association. Thyroid. 2009;19:565-612.
3. Rodriguez JM, Balsalobre M, Ponce JL, et al. Pheochromocytoma in MEN2A syndrome. Study of 54 patients. World J Surg. 2008;32:2520-6.

CHAPTER

23

Unusual Case of Hypoglycemia

Mini R Abraham

CASE PRESENTATION

Ms KC, a 45-year-old female, presented with history of hypoglycemic symptoms since her teenage years. There was no temporal relation to time of the day, physical activity, or meal. She started having more frequent symptoms for several years as an adult and was seen by different physicians including endocrinologists. She was evaluated to rule out insulinoma multiple times based on standard protocols but the diagnosis could not be made because of the lack of biochemical data suggestive of insulinoma. Patient also had multiple magnetic resonance imagings (MRIs) of pancreas done and reported negative. When first seen in our office, she reported two earlier serious episodes of hypoglycemia requiring assistance. One of those caused a motor vehicle accident also. Patient was seen in the emergency room on both occasions and there have been documentations of finger stick blood sugars in the 40–50 mg/dL ranges, but the rest of evaluations done on those occasions also failed to definitively establish diagnosis of insulinoma. Otherwise she reported symptoms of hypoglycemia at least two to three times per week. By now she had come up with her own plan to address the symptoms. She eats every 2–3 hours, and carries sugar tablets or candies with her all the time in case she becomes symptomatic. She noticed that she had been gaining weight. She was clearly overweight at the time of presentation. At one point, she was given metformin by one of her physicians thinking that this could be the "reactive hypoglycemia" which could happen in the early years of type-2 diabetes. Patient's physical examination was normal for blood pressure and other vitals. Her medications included simvastatin for high cholesterol and aspirin. Patient has been working full time and has been managing daily life and trying to address hypoglycemic symptoms.

Patient was advised to check blood sugar before treating herself with glucose. Patient was given a glucometer and she was instructed to check her finger stick blood sugar, whenever she would get symptoms. She documented few finger stick readings in the 50 mg/dL without any pattern, could be fasting or in between meals. She did not have symptoms all the time either. Patient also wore a continuous glucose monitor for about 5 days and these documented interstitial sugars in the 40–50 mg/dL range on several occasions. We were not able to document the low blood sugar with a venous blood draw to help meet the Whipple's triad for diagnosis of insulinoma. Another MRI obtained at a local imaging facility was reported negative and without any abnormality in the pancreas. Patient continued to have symptoms and she received a personal glucose sensor that she started to wear all the time.

HOSPITAL COURSE

- To explore further, patient was admitted to hospital where following laboratory data was generated:
    - Fasting plasma glucose: 60 mg/dL
    - Fasting plasma cortisol: 8 μg/dL
    - Cortrosyn-stimulated cortisol at 30 minutes: 23 μg/dL and 60 minutes cortisol of 28 μg/dL
    - Drug screen for sulfonylurea and nonsulfonylurea secretogauges: Negative.
- *Mixed meal test* (she had an apple, 6 almonds, and a fiber protein bar for the mixed meal test):
    - Fasting plasma glucose of 42 mg/dL with a corresponding insulin level of 10.3 μIU/mL and C-peptide level of 1.4 ng/mL
    - During her mixed meal test her plasma glucose dropped to 19 mg/dL in 60 minutes and patient was asymptomatic. Plasma C-peptide level at that time was 1.6 ng/mL, insulin level was not reported
- *72-hour fast:* After 19 hours of fast, her blood sugar dropped to 34 mg/dL with a concomitant insulin level at 4.8 μIU/mL and a C-peptide level of 1.3 ng/mL. She was given intravenous glucagon at the end of fast and this caused an increase in plasma glucose from 34 to 76 mg/dL. Beta hydroxybutyrate was also low at 0.3 when her plasma glucose was 34 mg/dL. Patient had reported blurry vision and the staff noticed decreased alertness and slight confusion when the blood sugar was 34 mg/dL
- *Computed tomography (CT) scan without and with intravenous (IV) contrast enhancement* with biphasic imaging of pancreas. There was a 1.8 × 1.3 cm hyper enhancing mass in the pancreatic body with imaging features typical for an islet cell tumor
- *Selective pancreatic arterial calcium injection (SPACI)*: There was >10-fold increase in her insulin levels after calcium gluconate injection of the superior mesenteric artery and negative results were found on splenic and gastroduodenal artery, and therefore based on this test, the assumption

was that the patient most likely has a functioning insulinoma in the tail of the pancreas

- Patient was scheduled for surgery and had distal pancreatectomy and splenectomy. Intraoperative ultrasound examination of the pancreas showed the head and neck of the pancreas normal
- Pathology report: Pancreas with multiple an islet cell tumors. The largest tumor was 2.0 cm × 1.7 cm × 1.0 cm located 1.0 cm from the surgical resection margin. A second tumor was located 1.0 cm distal to the largest tumor and measured 0.8 cm × 0.8 cm × 0.7 cm. There were additional microadenomas present in random sections of the pancreas.

DISCUSSION

Historical Perspective

In 1923, Fletcher and Campbell were the first to describe excessive insulin administration as etiology for hypoglycemia. Wilder and his colleagues confirmed link between insulin and hypoglycemia, when they described a case of hypoglycemia caused by a malignant insulinoma. First resection of an Insulinoma took place in 1927 when a tumor was removed from a physician, and the tumor extract caused hypoglycemia when injected into a rabbit. In 1935, Whipple and Frantz identified 75 cases in their review of literature and added 6 surgically proven cases of their own. This lead to coinage of term "Whipple's triad" that comprises low blood glucose, symptoms of hypoglycemia, and relief by food to establish the diagnosis of a hypoglycemic disorder. By 1950, nearly 400 cases had been reported. This number has increased manifold now.

In 1938, Laidlaw introduced the term "nesidioblastosis" or diffuse hyperplasia of an islets as a cause for hypoglycemia. This condition is characterized by diffuse hypertrophy and hyperplasia of an islet cells. This condition can cause hypoglycemia in infants as a result of mutations in the sulfonylurea receptor (*SUR1*) or in the potassium channel (*Kir6.2*) genes. The condition can occur very rarely in adults without the mutation. Preoperative differentiation from an insulinoma can be difficult but is suggested by negative imaging studies, associated with nonrestricted increase in insulin concentration following SPACI.

Incidence

Insulinoma is a very rare disorder. Mayo clinic experience reports that the incidence in Olmsted County, Minnesota, was about eight cases per million patient years based on the observation from 1927 to 1986, but half of them were incidentally found at autopsy. A subsequent series from the same institution, 1987–2007, reported very similar observation in terms of age and gender distribution. Reports from other parts of the world yield an incidence of about 1–2 cases/million patient years. The incidence of adult onset nesidioblastosis would be expected to be only about 0.3 cases per million patient years. Insulinomas have been observed in all ethnic groups.

Demographics

Insulinoma occurs more frequently in women than in men. The median age at onset is 45 years and most patients have been between 30 and 70 years of age. It is uncommon in individuals older than 80 years. Only few cases of childhood insulinomas have been reported.

Pathophysiology

The hypoglycemia in insulinoma is due to dysregulated insulin release. Normally increased plasma insulin and, hypoglycemia both suppress further insulin release. In insulinoma patients, suppression of insulin release by insulin and hypoglycemia is impaired and the insulin release is described as chaotic, and often not appropriately increased by hyperglycemia. Some patients may even present with abnormal glucose tolerance. Insulinoma is a neuroendocrine tumor, derived primarily from pancreatic an islet cells. About 90% of insulinomas are benign. Ten percent of insulinomas are malignant. About 10% have multiple insulinomas, and among these, 50% have multiple endocrine neoplasia type 1 (MEN1). Otherwise insulinomas are associated with MEN1 in 5% of cases. About 20% of patients with MEN1 develop insulinomas. Patients and their family members should be screened for MEN1.

Symptoms and Signs

Symptoms result from hypoglycemia and manifest as those related to sympathetic nervous system activation (sympatho-adrenal symptoms), and those related to neural deprivation of glucose (neuroglycopenic symptoms). The neuroglycopenic symptoms include confusion, visual change, dysarthria, seizures, and unusual behavior. Sympatho-adrenal symptoms include palpitations, diaphoresis, and shakiness. The time between the onset of symptoms and the diagnosis is about 3–5 years. There are case reports of patients, who had been symptomatic for decades before getting diagnosed with insulinoma. Many patients had initial diagnoses of epilepsy, depression, or psychoneurosis.

Patients with MEN1 may have symptoms from associated hormone hypersecretion such as hyperparathyroidism or other excess hormone secretions such as gastrin, vasoactive intestinal peptide, or adrenocorticotropic hormone (ACTH).

The physical examination is usually normal except in patients with malignant insulinoma in whom abdominal mass or signs of metastasis could be present.

DIFFERENTIAL DIAGNOSIS

Given that hypoglycemia emerged first during adulthood, hyperinsulinemia of infancy can be excluded right away. Diagnosis should include considerations that apply to hypoglycemia encountered in adults. Therefore, following conditions deserve to be taken into account:

- Iatrogenic: Related to surreptitious use of insulin, and insulin secretagogue (sulfonylureas and nonsulfonylurea drugs)
- Nesidioblastosis:
  - De novo
  - Described in patients with the postgastric bypass hypoglycemia
- Insulinoma
- Insulin autoimmune hypoglycemia in patients with antibodies directed against endogenous insulin or the insulin receptor
- Chronic illness: Hepatic/renal disease.

A careful medication history must be taken. Since, self-medication is often found in those with easy access to medicines, medical, and paramedical personnel remain high suspects for self-medication with insulin or insulin secretagogue. Establishing diagnosis requires having a reliable insulin assay that is capable of detecting newer insulin analogs as well.

DIAGNOSIS

The diagnosis is established by the demonstration of inappropriately high insulin concentrations during a spontaneous or induced episode of hypoglycemia such as in a 72-hour fast or following a mixed meal test. The Gold standard remains the classic 72-hour fast. Hypoglycemia will develop in almost all insulinoma patients during this test. This should be conducted in a hospital setting under supervised conditions. The prolonged supervised fast is recommended to confirm that hypoglycemia is the cause of the symptom and reversing it relieves the symptom and also to assess the role of insulin in causing the hypoglycemia. Successful completion of a 72-hour fast without the occurrence of a hypoglycemic episode could rule out a serious hypoglycemic disorder except for nesidioblastosis. Many patients with nesidioblastosis may have a normal 72-hour fast test, and the only biochemical abnormality may be postprandial hypoglycemia associated with increase in the plasma insulin and C-peptide level. This explains why the 72-hour fast should begin after a standard meal.

Diagnosis must fulfill the following conditions:

1. Plasma glucose <50 mg/dL
2. Fasting plasma insulin >6 μIU/mL
3. Elevated C-peptide >2.5 ng/mL
4. Absence of sulfonylurea, nonsulfonylurea insulin secretagogue
5. Proinsulin >25% of insulin immunoreactivity
6. Suppression of serum β-hydroxybutyrate.

Fasting insulin (μIU/mL) to plasma glucose (mg/dL) ratio in fasting state may be of diagnostic help. Healthy people have a ratio of <0.25. The ratio increases in patients with insulinoma. Obese people may have a slightly increased ratio.

In ancillary tests such as secretin stimulation test [following administration of secretin (2 units/kg body weight], plasma insulin rises >200% in healthy individuals whereas in patients harboring Insulinoma production of insulin by healthy β cells is suppressed. This test is no longer in vogue. Similarly, C-peptide suppression test following infusion of hog insulin is also not in vogue either. This test takes advantage of the fact that in healthy individual insulin suppresses its own secretion. Exogenous insulin will suppress insulin from healthy β-cells but not from insulinoma. Modified hyperinsulinemic, eu- and hypo-glycemic clamp using lispro-insulin has been used to detect low levels of autonomous insulin secretion in small insulinomas.

Tumor localization: Once the diagnosis is made with the biochemical evaluation, imaging techniques are used to localize the tumor.

Noninvasive imaging studies:

1. Spiral CT scan
2. Magnetic resonance imaging
3. Transabdominal ultrasonography
4. Somatostatin receptor scintigraphy (Octreoscan)
5. Glucagon-like peptide-1 (GLP-1) receptor scintigraphy. This may be useful in octreoscan negative cases.

Invasive tests:

1. *Endoscopic ultrasonography*: In the Mayo Clinic series of insulinoma patients, the sensitivity of endoscopic ultrasound for localization of insulinoma was 75%.
2. *Selective pancreatic arterial injection of calcium*: This test is based on the observation that calcium stimulates the release of insulin from hyperfunctioning cells such as insulinomas or nesidioblastosis but not from normal β-cells. The test involves selective injection of calcium gluconate into the gastroduodenal, splenic, and the superior mesenteric arteries with the sampling of venous blood for insulin. The sensitivity of selective arterial calcium stimulation for localization of insulinoma was 93–95% in the Mayo Clinic series.

Treatment

Surgical removal of the insulinoma is the treatment of choice. The extent of the surgery depends on the size, location, and nature of the tumor such as in MEN1 with possibility of frequent multiple tumors.

1. Enucleation of the insulinoma
2. Partial distal pancreatectomy
3. Pancreaticoduodenectomy
4. Whipple procedure: Removal of the head of the pancreas, gastrectomy, duodenectomy, and splenectomy
5. Subtotal pancreatectomy.

Risk of recurrence: In the Mayo Clinic series for 196 patients from 1927 to 1986, 11 patients had recurrent hypoglycemia. The recurrences occurred from 4 to 18.5 years after the initial operation and the cumulative incidence of recurrence was 6% at 10 years and 8% at 20 years.

The overall survival rate of patient's with insulinoma did not differ from that in the general population. Patients with malignant insulinoma had slightly worse survival rate.

Medical Therapy

Medical therapy should be considered in patients who are not candidates for surgery, who refuse surgery and who have unresectable metastatic disease:

1. *Diazoxide:* This is given as 100–200 mg three times daily and this inhibits insulin secretion. More than half of patients with benign disease could be kept asymptomatic on this regimen. The main side effects include fluid retention and hirsutism. Thiazide diuretics can be used to treat the fluid retention.

2. *Octreotide*: This somatostatin analog has been found to be effective in some patients by inhibiting the secretion of insulin. This medicine has to be injected.
3. *Lanreotide*: This is another somatostatin analog that appears to have similar clinical efficacy as octreotide and is also available in a long-acting depot form (lanreotide-SR).
4. *Glucocorticoids, calcium channel blockers* (verapamil), and *phenytoin* have also been used with some success.
5. There are some data to suggest that refractory cases may respond to treatment with *everolimus*, an inhibitor of the mammalian target of rapamycin (*mTOR*).

Radiation Therapy

Experience with external beam radiotherapy in the treatment of an islet cell tumors is only limited. There are case reports which suggest that radiation therapy can be used as palliative therapy in patients who are not candidates for surgical resection.

Therapy for Metastatic Disease

1. The liver and regional lymph nodes are the most common sites of metastatic disease.
2. *Hepatic resection*: This is considered in patients with a limited number of hepatic metastases.
3. *Hepatic artery embolization*: This is also considered in patients as palliative measure in those who are not candidates for surgical resection. Liver metastases derive most of their blood supply from the hepatic artery, whereas the healthy hepatocytes derive their blood supply from the portal vein. This is the rationale for therapeutic embolization of the hepatic artery with the goal of inducing necrosis of the metastases without damaging the normal liver cells.
4. *Radiofrequency ablation, cryoablation*, and *radioembolization* are other approaches used to treat hepatic lesions.
5. *Liver transplantation*: This is considered investigational at this time.
6. *Chemotherapy*: Malignant insulinomas respond poorly to chemotherapy. The traditional regimen of choice includes streptozotocin and doxorubicin. The orally active alkylating agent temozolomide has also been used.
7. *Case in context*: Patient did well postoperatively with complete resolution of hypoglycemic episodes and hypoglycemic symptoms. Surgery was done 4 years ago and her most recent HbA1c was 6.2% and without any

pharmacotherapy. Three interesting features stand out. *First,* patient did not have fasting hypoglycemia to meet the diagnostic cutoff. *Second,* patient demonstrated postprandial hypoglycemia. Both these features are known characteristics of some patients with nesidioblastosis. *Third,* histological features were consistent with multiple adenomatosis rather than true nesidioblastosis. However, in literature, one finds the terms multiple adenomatosis and nesidioblastosis being used interchangeably.

KEY POINTS

- Hypoglycemia is frequently encountered as a result of insulin or insulin secretagogue use. However, it is a serious diagnosis when encountered in nondiabetic patients who are not likely to be using insulin or any drug with potential to increase endogenous insulin output. Approach to such patients needs to be carefully designed to determine underlying etiology in a cost-effective manner
- Possible confounders in the interpretation of acquired data help in offering speedy and effective treatment
- The 72-hour fast must be undertaken under strict medical supervision
- Newer modalities in imaging are helpful in those where routine imaging studies are negative, but where there is high index of suspicion, and biochemical data to support an organic pathology
- Surgery offers a definitive cure in patients with insulinoma (often benign)
- Patients and their family members should be screened for MEN1.

SUGGESTED READINGS

1. Chon S, Choi MC, Lee YJ, et al. Autoimmune hypoglycemia in patients with characterization of insulin receptor autoantibodies. Diabetes Metab J. 2011;35:80-5.
2. Hamdy O. Hypoglycemia. Medscape. 2014.
3. Hirshberg B, Cochran C, Skarulis MC, et al. Malignant insulinoma: spectrum of unusual clinical features. Cancer. 2005;104:264.
4. Pereira PL, Roche AJ, Maier GW, et al. Insulinoma and islet cell hyperplasia: value of the calcium intra-arterial stimulation test when findings of other preoperative studies are negative. Radiology. 1998;206:703.
5. Romeo S, Milione M, Gatti A, et al. Complete clinical remission and disappearance of liver metastases after treatment with somatostatin analogue in a 40-year old woman with a malignant insulinoma positive for somatostatin receptors type 2. Horm Res. 2006;65:120.
6. Service JF. Diagnostic approach to adults with hypoglycemic disorders. Endocrinol Metab Clin North Am. 1999;28:519-32.
7. Service JF. Insulinoma. 2014.

CHAPTER

24

Ectopic Adrenocorticotropic Hormone Syndrome

Mandip S Rawla, Romesh Khardori

CASE PRESENTATION

Patient is a 56-year-old African American male who was admitted for persistent abdominal pain. Abdominal computed tomography (CT) scan at the time showed a 5.3 cm × 5.2 cm × 4.2 cm mass in his pancreas (Fig. 24.1). Endoscopic ultrasound was performed which demonstrated a 3 cm mass with splenic artery compression. The patient underwent subtotal pancreatectomy and splenectomy with tumor staining positive for gastrin, focal positive for somatostatin, and glucagon, negative for insulin and negative for adrenocorticotropic hormone. Final pathology was consistent with a well-differentiated endocrine carcinoma, mostly likely gastrinoma (Figs 24.2 and 24.3). Serum gastrin level at the time was 734 pg/mL (normal: 0–115 pg/mL). Serum cortisol level was 11.3 µg/dL (normal: 6.2–19.4 µg/dL). The CT scan obtained earlier did not show any metastatic disease. He was discharged on pantoprazole 40 mg daily.

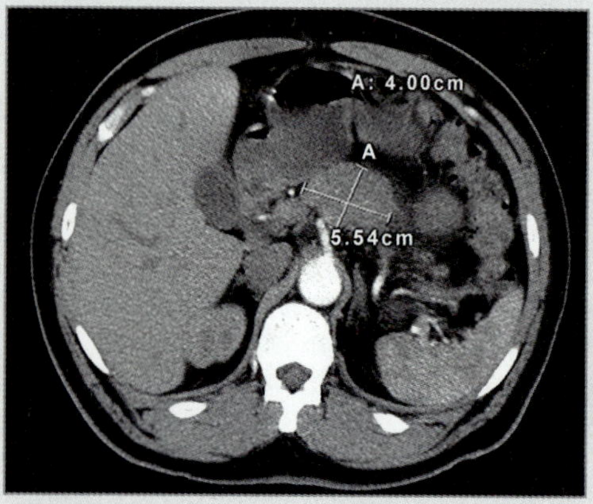

Figure 24.1: Pancreatic mass prior to resection

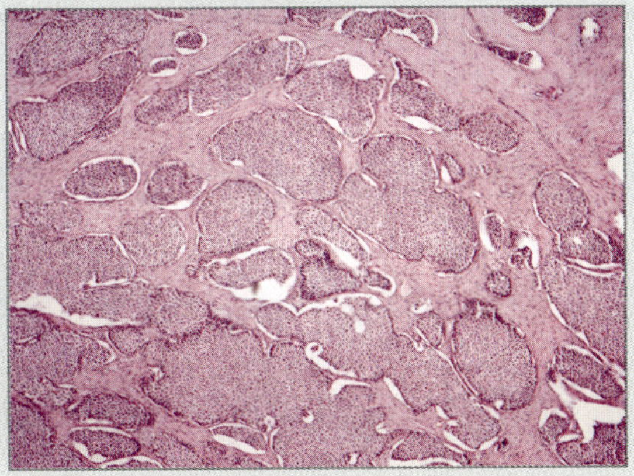

Figure 24.2: Gastrinoma: Low power

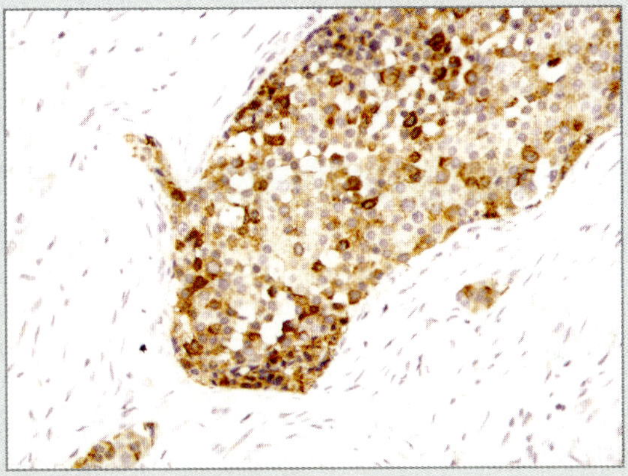

Figure 24.3: Gastrinoma: Immunoperoxidase stain

One year later, the patient was admitted for abdominal pain and diarrhea and was found to have evidence of disease recurrence with hepatic masses on CT scan. A serotonin level was checked as carcinoid was in the differential diagnosis because of history of chronic diarrhea. Serotonin level was 446 ng/mL (normal: 21–321 ng/mL), pancreatic polypeptide was 2042.6 pg/mL (normal: 0–418 pg/mL) and gastrin level was 6463 pg/mL. He was started on somatostatin (Sandostatin) treatment and maintained on high-dose protein pump inhibitors. By now he had new onset diabetes mellitus and was started on insulin. Later imaging demonstrated growth of the hepatic lesions and whole body metaiodobenzylguanidine (^{131}I-MIBG) scan was positive (Fig. 24.4). The patient underwent radio-embolization followed by chemoembolization of the hepatic masses and was started on tyrosine kinase inhibitor (sunitinib) by his oncologist.

With the exception of hand foot syndrome from sunitinib requiring dose reduction, the patient remained stable for about 2 more years. He was then admitted for shortness of breath, severe edema, and orthopnea refractory to outpatient diuretic management.

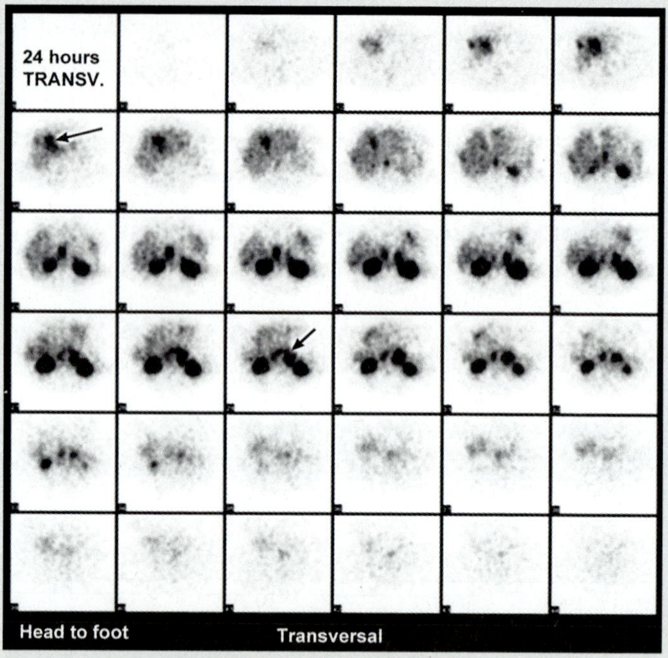

Figure 24.4: Positive octreotide scan. Arrows highlight the area of the liver metastasis and retroperitoneal lymphadenopathy

On examination, blood pressure was 183/94 mmHg with heart rate of 95 beats/minute. Examination revealed crackles bilaterally and 4 + bilateral pitting edema. Skin examination was significant for flushed appearance, abdominal striae, numerous skin tags, and acanthosis of the axilla.

DIFFERENTIAL DIAGNOSIS

Given his presentation with anasarca, consideration was given to congestive heart failure as well as renal failure. Investigations, however, were pertinent for normal heart function with an ejection fraction of 60% on echocardiogram, normal renal function with a serum creatinine of 0.8 mg/dL, without any proteinuria.

His physical examination findings of hypertension, abdominal striae and flushed appearance raised suspicion for Cushing's syndrome. Differential diagnosis with suspected Cushing's syndrome should include ectopic ACTH syndrome (EAS), Cushing's disease, and primary adrenal tumor. Other important consideration includes exogenous glucocorticoid use.

PERTINENT INVESTIGATIONS

Given negative initial work-up for his edema and shortness of breath and suspicion for Cushing's syndrome, additional testing was initiated. Work-up included:

- Random cortisol: 55.1 µg/dL (normal: 6.2–19.4 µg/dL) at 8 AM with a concurrent ACTH of 267.1 pg/mL (normal: 17.2–63.3 pg/mL)
- Midnight cortisol: 39.6 mg/dL demonstrating lack of circadian variation
- 24-hour urine cortisol: 1,945 µg/24 h (normal: 0–50 µg/24 h)
- Magnetic resonance imaging of the pituitary showed no tumor.

A high-dose dexamethasone suppression test was performed which showed lack of suppression of serum cortisol with a baseline level of 39.6 mg/dL prior to dexamethasone and a cortisol level of 35.6 µg/dL upon completion of the test. A 24 hour urine cortisol at the time of completion was also 1,123 mg/24 h. Of note, ACTH level remained high: 259 pg/mL. These data are consistent with ectopic ACTH secretion.

Selective venous sampling was pursued to further substantiate the diagnosis of ectopic ACTH secretion and to evaluate the potential source. Peripheral ACTH value was 282.6 pg/mL. Catheter sampling of the high right internal jugular vein showed an ACTH value of 290 pg/mL and high left internal jugular vein level was 305.2 pg/mL. The ratio therefore was 1.07 ruling out Cushing's disease and strongly favoring diagnosis of ectopic ACTH. Transhepatic venous sampling failed to reveal a gradient across liver.

MANAGEMENT

Treatment was initiated. Since there was no venous gradient on the ACTH venous sampling particularly within the hepatic veins, no primary tumor could be clearly identified. General surgery was consulted for consideration for bilateral adrenalectomy but our patient was deemed a poor surgical candidate. Therefore, ketoconazole, an imidazole, was started and increased to 200 mg three times daily. The patient developed transaminitis (*elevated AST and ALT*) within a few weeks so therapy had to be stopped. Metyrapone, an inhibitor of glucocorticoid synthesis (*inhibits 11β-hydroxylase*), was then started at 250 mg every 8 hours. Over a period of one month, this was titrated to a dose of 1,500 mg every 8 hours.

Despite dose escalation, hypercortisolemia persisted. Serum cortisol remained elevated at 40.7 mg/dL and urine cortisol was 638 mg/24 h. Next mitotane (o,p'DDD) was added. It was started at 500 mg every 8 hours and was titrated over 2 weeks to 1,500 mg every 8 hours. Urine-free cortisol was then used to monitor response to therapy, since, mitotane causes increase in cortisol-binding globulin making serum cortisol levels difficult to interpret.

Imaging by his oncologist showed persistent and enlarging right hepatic lobe metastasis and further chemoembolization was pursued. With this procedure along with aggressive medical therapy, patient demonstrated improvement in his blood glucose control, potassium levels; and his cortisol decreased from 42 to 16 µg/dL and urine cortisol improved from 638 to 91 mg/24 h. Treatment with mifepristone (RU-486) was also tried at 200 mg three times daily but limited availability of this medication limited its use. Soon afterward, he developed significant hypokalemia, which was managed with potassium replacement and high-dose spironolactone.

Over the next several months, the patient's outpatient course was complicated by his limited ability to pay for some of his maintenance medications. In addition, he had several readmissions to the hospital. Unfortunately, our patient's disease process persisted with recurrent hypercortisolemia despite attempts at aggressive medical management. Further his metastatic disease with hepatic lesions remained despite chemotherapy and embolization. Unfortunately, the patient succumbed to sepsis and pulmonary embolism.

DISCUSSION

Brown first alluded to ectopic secretory hormone state in 1928 when he described a patient with known oat cell carcinoma of the lung who presented with hyperpigmentation, diabetes, hirsutism, and muscle weakness. By 1961 over 40 well documented cases of hyperadrenocorticism associated with nonendocrine tissue tumors were described. In 1961, it was established that both plasma as well tumors of such patients contained a substance with biologic activity that was indistinguishable from that of ACTH. The term "ectopic ACTH syndrome" was later introduced by Liddle et al.

Ectopic ACTH syndrome is characterized by uncontrolled overproduction of ACTH by a nonpituitary source subsequently leading to hypercortisolism and presenting clinically as a frank Cushingoid state. Cushing symptoms include rapid weight gain particularly of the trunk and face, hyperhidrosis, purple striae, baldness, thinning of the skin, hirsutism, and proximal muscle weakness.

About 10–15% cases of Cushing's syndrome are due to ectopic ACTH secretion. Most common causes of ectopic ACTH production include small cell carcinoma of the lung, carcinoid tumors (most commonly of the lung), and neuroendocrine tumors. Most likely mechanism of uncontrolled ACTH production is disordered transactivation of pro-opiomelanocortin (POMC) in nonpituitary tissues. The POMC promoter is ordinarily methylated, and thus silenced, in most tissues except the pituitary gland. In tumors such as small cell lung carcinoma of the lung, demethylation occurs through oncogene activation leading to ectopic transcription and translation of the POMC in tumor cells. This results in overproduction of POMC, which in turn gets processed to ACTH. This further leads to uncontrolled hypercortisolism via downstream action. Unless specifically looked for, it may be missed in tissue immunohistochemistry studies.

When there is clinical suspicion of hypercortisolism, there are a number of diagnostic tests that can be performed. These include midnight serum cortisol level, midnight salivary cortisol level, and 24-hour urine-free cortisol excretion, and low-dose overnight dexamethasone suppression test. Random cortisol and ACTH levels should not be used in the work-up. Typically if the initial test is abnormal then a second test is performed to confirm the hypercortisolemic state.

Once the diagnosis is established, the focus then turns to finding the cause such as pituitary driven Cushing's disease or an EAS. Pertinent tests include the high-dose dexamethasone suppression test, corticotrophin-releasing hormone test, and inferior petrosal sinus sampling. Important radiographic studies include pituitary MRI and CT scan of the adrenals. If an occult EAS is suspected, CT or MRI of the chest, abdomen, and pelvis may be warranted. As in our patient with a known neuroendocrine tumor, an octreotide scan may be particularly useful. Neuroendocrine tumors have somatostatin receptors and are detected by administrating a radiolabeled analog of somatostatin. In our institution, indium 111-labeled octreotide is used.

The treatment of the EAS depends on the ability to locate the source or cause of excessive secretion. If a clear source can be determined, surgery is the treatment of choice. In the case of known malignancy such as small cell lung cancer, treatment may be limited to treatment of the malignancy itself. Bilateral adrenalectomy should be considered as well.

If surgery is not an option, as in our patient who was not deemed to be an acceptable surgical candidate, then medical treatment becomes the focus. Our patient is an excellent illustration of the number of drugs that can be used to suppress hypercortisolism (Table 24.1).

Ketoconazole is an imidazole and is most commonly used as an antifungal. It also works at several levels to block cortisol biosynthesis and additionally is an inhibitor of C17–20 desmolase, thus decreasing testosterone production. Usually 400–800 mg is needed to control hypercortisolism. An important side effect to monitor for with this agent is abnormal liver function tests. In our patient, there is limited use of this

TABLE 24.1: Medical treatment

Medication	Mechanism	Side effects
Ketoconazole	Blocks cytochrome p-450 dependent enzymes in the steroid pathway	Abnormal liver function tests, nausea, vomiting, headache, decreased libido
Metyrapone	Inhibits 11β-hydroxylase	Nausea, salt retention, hypertension
Mitotane (o,p'DDD)	Acts on adrenocortical cell mitochondria to block 11β-hydroxylase and results in necrosis of the adrenocortical cell	Nausea, fatigue, skin rash, neurotoxicity
Mifepristone	Glucocorticoid receptor antagonist	Nausea, vomiting, headache

agent. Other side effects to be aware of include nausea, vomiting, headache, decreased libido, and impotence.

Metyrapone inhibits 11β-hydroxylase and thus blocks the final step in cortisol biosynthesis. The dose can range from 250 mg four times daily to up to 6 g total per day. Drug effectiveness is monitored by serum and urine cortisol levels. Side effects include hirsutism, salt retention and hypertension. It is often used as an adjuvant to other drug therapy.

Mitotane (o,p'DDD) is an adrenolytic agent and is often used to perform a "medical adrenalectomy" in patients. It is frequently used in adrenal carcinomas. It acts on adrenocortical cell mitochondria to block 11β-hydroxylase and results in necrosis of the adrenocortical cell. It also reduces mineralocorticoid activity. Its effectiveness is long lasting and often glucocorticoid replacement is needed after prolonged use. Initial dose is 0.5 mg daily in the evening with dose titration up to 2–3 g daily. It is important to note that mitotane increases cortisol binding globulin thus causing an increase in total serum cortisol levels. As such, therapeutic response is monitored with 24 hour urine cortisol levels. Patients frequently report nausea and vomiting with the use of this agent.

Mifepristone or RU-486 is best known for its use in pregnancy termination but has also been approved by the Food and Drug Administration (FDA) for use in the management of hypercortisolism particularly in controlling hyperglycemia (FDA February 18, 2012). It has antiprogesterone effects but at high doses is a glucocorticoid receptor antagonist. Since it works as a receptor blocker rather than an inhibitor of production, cortisol levels cannot be used to determine effectiveness of treatment. Symptoms are typically followed. It is particularly effective at improving cortisol induced psychosis as well as glycemic control. Hypokalemia is a common side effect. Other side effects include nausea, vomiting, fatigue, and headache.

CONCLUSION

Medical therapy of EAS is challenging as illustrated in our patient. The medications used have several side effects and are often needed in combination to achieve reduction in hypercortisolism. Response to therapy needs to be monitored regularly with serum and urine cortisol levels. In addition, once these levels normalize, and symptoms improve, replacement glucocorticoid therapy should be initiated.

KEY POINTS

- Ectopic ACTH syndrome should be suspected in rapidly evolving Cushing's syndrome in setting of nonpituitary neoplasm
- Ectopic ACTH hormone may result from ectopic transactivation of POMC, or secretion of corticotropin-releasing hormone (CRH) or ACTH
- In presence of hepatic metastases, transarterial chemoembolization, or transarterial embolization can be considered. Local resection or radiofrequency ablation may be an option for oligonodular disease
- In presence of hepatic metastases, prognosis is poor
- Medical therapy may be chosen from a menu of medications currently available to offer palliation.

SUGGESTED READINGS

1. Illias I, Torpy DJ, Pacek K, et al. Cushing's syndrome due to ectopic corticotropin secretion: twenty years' experience at the National Institutes of Health. J Clin Endocrinol Metab. 2005;90:4955-62.
2. Liddle GW, Givens JR, Wendell G, et al. The Ectopic ACTH Syndrome. Cancer Res. 1965;25:1057-61.
3. Lin H-W, Tseng F-Y. Ectopic adrenalcorticotropic hormone syndrome improved by transarterial embolization to hepatic metastatic lesions of pancreatic neuroendocrine carcinoma: a case report. J Clin Oncol. 2012;30(33):e360-3.

CHAPTER

25 ACTH-Independent, Cushing's Syndrome Secondary to Primary-pigmented Nodular Adrenal Hyperplasia Associated with Carney's Complex

Celine Chaya, Joseph A Aloi

CASE PRESENTATION

A 16-year-old female was evaluated elsewhere for obesity, weight gain, and excessive facial hair growth. Her weight was 86 kg, blood pressure (BP) 130/80 mmHg. She had abdominal striae and a dorsal fat pad on physical examination. She denied use of any exogenous steroids. She was found to have nonsuppressible hypercortisolism.

Specifically, plasma cortisol concentration at 8:00 AM, following 1 mg dexamethasone administered at 11:00 PM the previous night, was 32.7 µg/dL. DHEA-S was 0.3 µg/mL (normal 0.3–2.9 µg/mL). Repeat dexamethasone suppression test (DST) with long low dose (0.5 mg Q6H for 2 days) failed to demonstrate cortisol suppression. Computed tomography (CT) scan of the sella and chest X-ray were normal. CT of the abdomen demonstrated mildly diffuse enlargement of the adrenal glands. She was treated for presumptive Cushing's disease with pituitary irradiation (45 Gy) and subsequently improved and felt to have an initial clinical response. Her weight decreased by 5 kg and abdominal striae became less prominent.

Four years later she was admitted to hospital at 24 weeks gestation with 20 kg weight gain, hypertension, and pretibial edema. Her weight was 104 kg, BP 160/100 mmHg. She had moon facies, diffuse upper thoracic and facial acne, facial hirsutism, dorsal and supraclavicular fat pads, thin friable skin, proximal muscle weakness, and severe pretibial edema.

Laboratory results on admission revealed: hypokalemia (potassium: 2.9–3.3 mEq/L), urinary protein excretion of 700 µg/24 h, normal thyroid function tests and an elevated fasting blood glucose of 159 mg/dL and urine-free cortisol of 2,700 µg/24 h. A high-dose DST was performed twice by administration of 2 mg every 6 hours for 48 hours, results in Table 25.1. Serum adrenocorticotropic hormone (ACTH) was consistently unmeasurable.

TABLE 25.1: Basal and post-HDST serum cortisol and 24-hour urine-free cortisol

	Serum cortisol (μg/dL)	Urine-free cortisol μg/24 h (Normal <100 μg/24 h)
Basal (Test 1)	52.3	2,700
Basal (Test 2)	43.9	2,233
High DST (Test 1)	47.2	2,690
High DST (Test 2)	59	3,128

DIFFERENTIAL DIAGNOSIS

Cushing's syndrome (CS) phenotype with key hormonal abnormalities similar to an established case of CS may be seen in flowing situations:

- Polycystic ovarian syndrome (PCOS)
- Uncontrolled diabetes mellitus (type 2)
- Pseudo-CS
- Primary generalized glucocorticoid resistance
- Metabolic syndrome.

According to the evidence-based 2008 Endocrine Society Clinical Guidelines, one of the following initial tests is recommended for diagnosis of CS:

- Urine-free cortisol (at least two measurements)
- Late-night salivary cortisol (two measurements)
- 1-mg overnight DST
- Longer low-dose DST (2 mg/day for 48 hours).

With an elevated 24-hour urine-free cortisol level tested twice, the diagnosis of CS was made in our patient.

After the diagnosis of hypercortisolism is established, its cause must be determined.

- The first step in the evaluation is to determine whether it is ACTH-dependent or ACTH-independent by measuring plasma ACTH.

ACTH-dependent causes

- Cushing's disease (pituitary)
- Ectopic ACTH syndrome
- Ectopic corticotropin-releasing hormone (CRH) syndrome
- Macronodular adrenal hyperplasia
- Iatrogenic (treatment with natural or synthetic ACTH).

ACTH-independent causes

- Adrenal adenoma
- Adrenal carcinoma
- Primary-pigmented nodular adrenocortical disease (PPNAD) and Carney's syndrome
- Massive macronodular adrenocortical disease
- McCune–Albright syndrome
- Iatrogenic (steroid administration)
- Macronodular adrenal hyperplasia.

The patient's ACTH was <5 pg/mL (normal: 10–60 pg/mL). The suppressed ACTH concentration constitutes strong evidence in favor of ACTH-independent CS (to be noted that at the time of the initial presentation assays for ACTH measurement were not readily available).

- The next step in diagnosis is imaging of the adrenal glands.

CT of the abdomen did show prominent adrenal glands without nodules that make carcinoma, adenoma, or macronodular hyperplasia less likely (Fig. 25.1). There was no history of steroid intake ruling out iatrogenic cause. She did not have the phenotypic presentation of McCune–Albright syndrome (*café-au-lait* macules and precocious puberty). She did in fact have a paradoxical increase in urine-free cortisol (UFC) after dexamethasone administration (as illustrated in Table 25.1), which is characteristic of PPNAD.

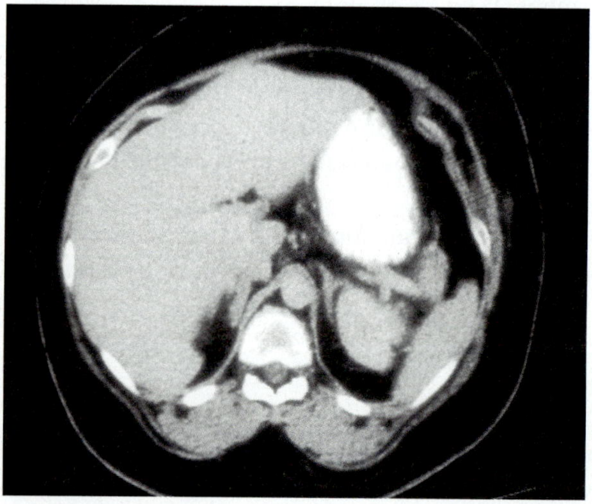

Figure 25.1: Abdominal CT with bilateral adrenal enlargement

MANAGEMENT

She was treated with *metyrapone* during pregnancy. Her clinical status rapidly improved with amelioration of facial acne, skin manifestations, and peripheral edema, as manifested by a decrease in weight from 102–97 kg over 4 days. Blood pressure and serum potassium normalized rapidly and antihypertensive medications and potassium supplements were discontinued. Urine-free cortisol on day 6 was 73 μg/day. The patient successfully delivered a healthy male infant.

She was reevaluated postpartum and underwent bilateral adrenalectomy. Findings were consistent with PPNAD. Macroscopic evaluation revealed multiple brownish nodules. Histologic sections showed multiple pigmented cortical nodules composed primarily of medium to large cells with abundant eosinophilic cytoplasm.

She underwent genetic screening that showed the presence of an inactivating mutation of the protein kinase cAMP-dependent regulatory type 1α (*PRKAR1α*) gene [*this gene codes for type1A regulatory subunit of protein kinase A* (PKA)], which along with PPNAD, fulfill the criteria for diagnosis of Carney's syndrome. Echocardiogram did not show atrial masses or myxoma. Her son underwent testing and was found to have a paradoxical increase in urinary cortisol after Liddle's test. Screening was recommended to all first-degree relatives but the rest of the family declined. Of note, the patient's mother has had excision of a left atrial mass, presumed a myxoma.

DISCUSSION

Primary-pigmented micronodular adrenal hyperplasia is an adrenocortical cause of CS. Cushing's syndrome due to bilateral adrenal lesions (micronodular and macronodular adrenal hyperplasia and bilateral adenomas or carcinomas) is seen in 10–15% cases. Micronodular adrenal hyperplasia is defined by the presence of multiple cortical micronodules measuring <1 cm in diameter. The PPNAD is characterized by multiple pigmented black or brown micronodules surrounded by areas of internodular cortical atrophy. This can be seen as a *string of beads* on thin-section high-resolution CT scan and the overall size of the adrenal gland is often not enlarged. Those micronodules secrete excess cortisol independently of ACTH stimulation.

Patients with PPNAD exhibit a paradoxical increase in cortisol secretion in response to administration of dexamethasone at doses of 2 mg/day for 2 days followed by 8 mg/day for 2 days (Liddle's test). A >50% increase in urinary free cortisol (UFC) excretion on the second day of high-dose dexamethasone administration compared with basal level usually supports the diagnosis of PPNAD. This abnormal cortisol response is now an accepted biological criterion for the diagnosis of the disease. The molecular mechanisms involved in dexamethasone-induced cortisol secretion are not fully elucidated. It is considered to be the consequence of activation of the cAMP/PKA pathway through glucocorticoid receptors which are present in the PPNAD micronodules. This paradoxical response has also been reported in nonpigmented bilateral micronodular adrenal hyperplasia with ectopic adrenal adenoma. However, PKA-mediated effect of dexamethasone could not be traced to glucocorticoid receptor suggesting nongenomic effect of dexamethasone through unknown membrane receptor (Louiset et al. 2010).

Our patient did have the paradoxical increase in cortisol suggestive of PPNAD. The diagnosis was eventually confirmed histologically after she underwent bilateral adrenalectomy. The PPNAD may be isolated or may occur as part of the Carney complex (CNC).

Carney Complex

The CNC was originally described by Carney et al. (1985) as "the complex of myxomas, spotty skin pigmentation, and endocrine over activity." It is classified as a multiple endocrine neoplasia syndrome, with affected patients having endocrine gland tumors, including adrenal (PPNAD), pituitary (GH and prolactinoma), testicular (Sertoli cell tumor), thyroid (follicular hyperplasia to carcinoma), and ovarian cysts. The most frequent endocrine manifestation of CNC is ACTH-independent CS caused by PPNAD.

In a 2010 publication, Almeida and Stratakis suggested the diagnostic criteria (Table 25.2) for CNC based on clinical, imaging, biochemical testing, and genetic studies.

Definite diagnosis of CNC requires two or more major manifestations. Diagnosis may also be made if one major criterion is present and a first-degree relative has CNC or an inactivating mutation of the gene encoding PKA regulatory subunit 1α (PRKAR1α). Our patient did have confirmed PPNAD, and an inactivating mutation of the *PRKAR1*α gene that fulfills the criteria for diagnosis of CNC.

Carney complex may be inherited as an autosomal dominant trait but in a significant number of patients the disease is sporadic, presumably due to de novo mutations. To date, three genetic loci associated with a predisposition to CNC have been reported (17q22-24 locus referred as CNC1; 2p16 locus referred as CNC2, and 17p12-13.1). To date four responsible genes have been identified: *PPKAR1A*, *PDE11A*, *PDE8B*, and *MYH8* (without adrenal involvement). The PDE11A and PDE8B mutations have been identified in nonpigmented forms of micronodular adrenal hyperplasia. Besides

TABLE 25.2: Diagnostic criteria for Carney complex

Major diagnostic criteria

- Spotty skin pigmentation with typical distribution (lips, conjunctiva and inner or outer canthi, vaginal, and penile mucosa)
- Myxoma* (cutaneous and mucosal)
- Cardiac myxoma*
- Breast myxomatosis* or fat-suppressed magnetic resonance imaging findings suggestive of this diagnosis
- PPNAD* or paroxical positive response of urinary glucocorticoid excretion to dexamethasone administration during Liddle's test
- Acromegaly due to GH-producing adenoma*
- LCCSCT* or characteristic calcification on testicular ultrasound
- Thyroid carcinoma* or multiple hypoechoic nodules on thyroid ultrasound in a young patient
- Psammomatous melanotic schwannomas*
- Blue nevus, epithelioid blue nevus*
- Breast ductal adenoma*
- Osteochondromyxoma*

Supplemental criteria

- Affected first-degree relative
- Inactivating mutation of the *PRKAR1α* gene

PPNAD, primary pigmented nodular adrenocortical disease; LCCSCT, large-cell calcifying Sertoli cell tumor; *PRKAR1α*: protein kinase A regulatory subunit 1α.

*After histological confirmation.

PRKAR1α mutations, somatic β-catenin mutations have been found in larger nodules of patients with PPNAD.

The *PRKAR1α* gene is located in CNC1 locus. The genes responsible for CNC at the CNC2 locus remain unknown. PRKAR1α mutations are present in up to 80% of the patients that present with CS associated with PPNAD. Protein kinase A is an important enzyme in cyclic adenosine monophosphate (c-AMP)-mediated endocrine signaling pathways. Altered PKA function leads to activation of the c-AMP/PKA pathway which is associated with multiple and autonomous endocrine tumors.

In a 2001 publication, Stratakis et al. suggested the following annual studies for patients with established CNC:

1. Echocardiogram
2. Measurement of UFC levels and serum IGF-I levels
3. Male patients should also have testicular ultrasonography at the initial evaluation; minute calcifications, presumably large-cell calcifying Sertoli cell tumor (LCCSCT), may be followed by annual ultrasound thereafter

4. Thyroid ultrasonography should be obtained at the initial evaluation, and may be repeated as needed
5. Transabdominal pelvic ultrasonography in female patients is recommended during the first evaluation but need not be repeated, unless there is a detectable abnormality, because of the low risk of ovarian malignancy
6. Breast imaging may be required for the detection of breast tumors.

Carney complex should not be confused with Carney triad that refers to constellation of gastric leiomyosarcoma, paraganglioma, and pulmonary chondroma. Recently a fourth component has been added to this triad namely, adrenal cortical adenoma (Carney 2013).

Hypokalemia and Cushing's Syndrome

Hypokalemia only rarely occurs with CS, it is secondary to very high levels of cortisol saturating the enzyme which usually degrades excess cortisol, allowing excess cortisol to bind to mineralocorticoid receptors with resultant hypokalemia. Interesting endocrine disorders associated with hypokalemia include pheochromocytoma, primary aldosteronism, and Liddle's syndrome.

Our patient's hypokalemia was difficult to correct. It resolved completely after medical treatment of CS.

Pregnancy and Cushing's Syndrome

Diagnosis of CS during pregnancy can be challenging. By third trimester, total plasma glucose, corticosteroid binding globulin (CBG) and 24-hour UFC rise threefold compared with healthy controls. Plasma-free cortisol increases 1.6-fold. Furthermore some commercial immunoassays overestimate UFC by 30–35% during pregnancy compared with liquid chromatography-mass spectrometry. Fetus is protected partially from maternal hypercortisolemia because of placental 11β-hydroxysteroid dehydrogenase that converts 85% of maternal cortisol to biologically inactive cortisone. Suppression of cortisol by dexamethasone is blunted particularly during second and the third trimester of pregnancy.

TREATMENT

Bilateral adrenalectomy is the recommended treatment for patients with CS associated with PPNAD or CNC. Medical treatment with adrenal enzyme inhibitors has been used to reduce cortisol secretion and improve the physical condition of patients with severe CS before adrenal surgery. Our patient was treated with metyrapone as an interim until definitive surgical treatment was feasible. Drugs like Ketoconazole and mitotane are best avoided during pregnancy. Mifepristone is clearly contraindicated during pregnancy. Treating CS appears to prevent stillborn deliveries, but does not affect frequency of intrauterine growth restriction or premature birth.

KEY POINTS

- Primary pigmented nodular adrenocortical disease is an ACTH-independent disorder resulting in CS. It is a rare disorder that is diagnosed in 1% cases. It occurs sporadically or may be as part of CNC or isolated PPNAD
- A mutation of PRKAR1α, a tumor suppressor gene, has been identified in more than half of CNC kindreds. Families that do not carry the PRKAR1α mutation are thought to map to the CNC2 locus and possibly other loci
- It is often difficult to distinguish PPNAD from other ACTH independent causes of CS since adrenal size is often not enlarged
- Sequential low-dose and high-dose DST helps in distinguishing PPNAD from other primary adrenocortical lesions because of paradoxical rise in UFC following dexamethasone administration seen in close to 75% of cases
- Screening for other tumors of Carney's complex should be performed
- Bilateral adrenalectomy is the recommended treatment of choice followed by lifelong glucocorticoid replacement.

SUGGESTED READINGS

1. Almeida MQ, Stratakis CA. Carney complex and other conditions associated with micronodular adrenal hyperplasias. Best Pract Res Clin Endocrinol Metab. 2010;24(6):907-14.
2. Handler J. Cushing's syndrome with uncontrolled hypertension, occasional hypokalemia and two pregnancies. J Clin Hypertension. 2010;12:516-21.
3. Lim WH, Torpy DJ, Jaffries WS. The medical management of Cushing's syndrome during pregnancy. Eur J Obstet Gynecol Rep Biol. 2013;168:1-6.
4. Louiset E, Stratakis CA, Perraudin V, et al. The paradoxical increase in cortisol secretion induced by dexamethasone in primary pigmented nodular adrenocortical disease involves glucocorticoid receptor-mediated effect of dexamethasone on protein kinase a catalytic subunit. J Clin Endocrinol Metab. 2009;94(7):2406-13.
5. Stratakis CA, Boikos SA. Genetics of adrenal tumors associated with Cushing's syndrome: a new classification for bilateral adrenocortical hyperplasias. Nat Clin Pract Endocrinol Metab. 2007;3(11):748-57.

CHAPTER

26

Vitamin D Toxicity

Parjeet Kaur, Sunil K Mishra, Ambrish Mithal

CASE PRESENTATION

A 78-year-old lady presented with a history of weakness, polyuria, intense thirst, difficulty in speaking and following commands, staggering walk, and confusion for the last 4 weeks. There was no history of fall, head injury, fever, headache, or any focal weakness. The patient's son reported that for last several months she had complaints of bone pain and difficulty in walking for which she was evaluated by her primary care physician. She was found to have low-serum 25 hydroxyvitamin D (25(OH)D = 12 ng/mL), normal serum calcium with serum creatinine of 1.6 mg/dL. She was treated for vitamin D deficiency with six injections of vitamin D3 (600,000 IU each) over a period of 1 month. She was diagnosed to have hypertension 10 years back and was well controlled on amlodipine 5 mg once daily. She had history of primary hypothyroidism and was taking levothyroxine 100 μg once daily. Past history revealed that she had undergone left nephrectomy because of nonfunctioning kidney.

On physical examination her blood pressure was 150/90 mmHg, the pulse rate 100/min and temperature 98.6°F. The patient was irritable. Her oral mucosa was dry. Cardiovascular, respiratory, and abdominal examination did not reveal any abnormality. There were no signs of focal neurological deficit.

INVESTIGATIONS

Initial laboratory evaluation showed

- Serum calcium: 14.8 mg/dL
- Phosphorus: 3.8 mg/dL
- Alkaline phosphatase: 120 IU/L
- Intact parathyroid hormone (iPTH): 198 pg/mL
- Serum vitamin D (25(OH)D): 378 ng/mL

- Serum 1,25 dihydroxy vitamin D (1,25(OH)$_2$D): Normal (30 pg/mL)
- Blood urea: 98 mg/dL
- Serum creatinine: 2.4 mg/dL
- Hemoglobin: 10.5 g/dL
- Total leucocyte count: 12,500/µL (mildly raised)
- Erythrocyte sedimentation rate (ESR) in the first hour: 10
- Serum sodium: 131 mEq/L
- Potassium: 4.4 mEq/L
- Liver function tests: Normal
- Serum albumin: 3.1 g/L
- Thyroid function test: showed suppressed thyroid-stimulating hormone (TSH) (0.156 mIU/mL) with high normal FT4–1.78 ng/dL
- Urine examination: 6–8 WBCs/hpf (white blood cells/high power field).

DIFFERENTIAL DIAGNOSIS

Hypercalcemia is broadly classified into PTH dependent (where iPTH levels are elevated) and PTH independent where iPTH levels are appropriately suppressed.

PTH-dependent hypercalcemia is seen in:

- Primary hyperparathyroidism
- Tertiary hyperparathyroidism
- Familial hypocalciuric hypercalcemia due to mutated calcium sensing receptor
- Hypercalcemia associated with lithium use
- Ectopic iPTH secretion (rare).

PTH-independent hypercalcemia is encountered in:

- Hypercalcemia of malignancy (humoral hypercalcemia)
- Vitamin D toxicity
- Granulomatous disorders such as sarcoidosis, tuberculosis, candidiasis, and berylliosis
- Hodgkin's lymphoma
- Thiazide induced hypercalcemia
- Vitamin A intoxication
- Milk alkali syndrome
- Hyperthyroidism
- Acromegaly, pheochromocytoma, adrenal insufficiency
- Prolonged immobilization.

Primary hyperparathyroidism and hypercalcemia of malignancy comprise >90% of cases of hypercalcemia. Raised iPTH levels in the presence of hypercalcemia in the aforementioned case suggest that the patient may have a PTH-dependent cause of hypercalcemia. However, detailed clinical history plays a significant role in diagnostic approach to hypercalcemia and history of intake of very high dose of vitamin D (3,600,000 IU) over a short period of 1 month in this patient makes the diagnosis of vitamin D toxicity highly likely. This was further supported by the presence of highly raised serum 25(OH)D level. The patient was also evaluated for possibilities of primary and tertiary hyperparathyroidism in view of raised iPTH. Sestamibi scan was obtained; no parathyroid abnormality was visualized. Serum creatinine was elevated in this patient that could be due to acute deterioration of kidney function caused by dehydration. However, possibility of chronic kidney disease cannot be ruled out as she had single kidney and her baseline serum creatinine (before receiving vitamin D) was also above the upper limit of normal. Finding of raised iPTH in the setting of vitamin D toxicity in this patient could be explained by presence of coexisting chronic kidney disease.

MANAGEMENT

The patient was admitted and managed in intensive care unit. Hypercalcemia was managed with intravenous fluids (0.9% w/v of NaCl) with careful monitoring of central venous pressure and intake/output as patient was elderly and had evidence of kidney disease. Glucocorticoids (intravenous hydrocortisone 50 mg 8 hourly for 1 week) and calcitonin (100 IU subcutaneous 8 hourly for 5 days) were also used to manage hypercalcemia. Bisphosphonates were not considered because of underlying kidney disease with a past history of nephrectomy. Her clinical symptoms including irritability improved with decline in serum calcium level. Serum calcium decreased to 9.2 mg/dL on day 3. Other parameters improved and serum creatinine declined to 1.6 mg/dL by day 5.

A final diagnosis of vitamin D toxicity with chronic kidney disease and secondary hyperparathyroidism was made. Levothyroxine dose was reduced to 75 μg once daily. She was discharged on day 8 with serum calcium of 8.8 mg/dL and instructions to maintain hydration and avoid calcium and vitamin D supplements. She was advised follow-up after 2 weeks with repeat serum calcium.

She was readmitted with history of fall, abnormal behavior, and raised calcium of 11.24 mg/dL, 1 month after discharge. She was managed conservatively and low dose zoledronate (2 mg) was administered intravenously. Hypercalcemia was corrected with no subsequent recurrence.

DISCUSSION

Vitamin D toxicity is almost always an iatrogenic problem and the case presented above is an illustration of an overzealous attempt to correct vitamin D deficiency. Vitamin D toxicity is a preventable entity and if undiagnosed can often be life threatening. Recent awareness regarding vitamin D deficiency and splurge in irrational use of vitamin D and calcium supplements has pushed this "uncommon cause of hypercalcemia" to "not so uncommon cause of hypercalcemia," in some geographical areas of the world like India.

Vitamin D toxicity can result from excess intake of vitamin D (oral or parenteral) or its analogs. Vitamin D is used therapeutically to treat certain hypocalcemic disorders such as osteomalacia, hypoparathyroidism, pseudohypoparathyroidism, and hypocalcemia associated with chronic renal disease. Improper use of pharmaceutical preparations of vitamin D is the most common cause of vitamin D toxicity. With the recent data showing widespread vitamin D deficiency even among healthy individuals and its association with various nonskeletal disorders, indiscriminate use of vitamin D has risen markedly in clinical practice especially to treat nonspecific back and leg pains that are presumed to be due to vitamin D deficiency. Vitamin D intoxication has also been described to occur with the use of over the counter supplements and even milk fortification. Moreover, there are reports of accidental consumption of very high doses of vitamin D. Vitamin D toxicity can occur in granulomatous diseases such as sarcoidosis by mechanism of excessive conversion of 25(OH)D to $1,25(OH)_2D$. Excessive sun exposure alone cannot result in vitamin D toxicity, since the additional ultraviolet B light leads to local inactivation of vitamin D3.

The maximum chronic daily oral intake of vitamin D that can be given safely without any adverse effects for most healthy adults has not been established. Most of the reports of vitamin D toxicity have documented vitamin D intake of >40,000 IU/day. The Food and Nutrition Board recommends the tolerable upper intake level (UL) as 1,000 IU daily for infants 0–6 months of age, 1,500 IU daily for infants 6–12 months of age, 2,500 IU daily for children 1–3 years of age, 3,000 IU daily for children 4–8 years of age, and 4,000 IU daily subsequently throughout life.

Vitamin D in its parent form is more lipophilic and therefore has longer half-life (20 days to months) as compared to its less lipophilic metabolites

25(OH)D and 1,25$(OH)_2$D that have relatively shorter half-life of 15 days (up to 2 months in studies with radiolabeled vitamin D) and 15–20 hours, respectively. Longer the half-life, longer is the duration of toxicity. Due to slow release of vitamin D from fat deposits, hypercalcemia secondary to parent vitamin D overdose can last up to 12–18 months even after dosing is discontinued. Susceptibility to vitamin D toxicity may be influenced by various factors including the concentration of the vitamin D metabolite, 1α-hydroxylase activity, vitamin D receptor (VDR) number, the capacity of the vitamin-D-binding protein (DBP), and the degradation pathway. Mechanism of vitamin D toxicity is explained by activation of VDR by vitamin D metabolites in the nucleus of target cells with subsequent amplification of gene expression. High plasma 25(OH)D levels in vitamin D toxicity exceed the DBP-binding capacity that in turn causes "free 25(OH)D" to enter the cell, where it acts directly on VDR and affect gene expression. The potent metabolite 1,25$(OH)_2$D has the least affinity for DBP. Following vitamin D overdose, concentrations of vitamin D, and its metabolites rise that exceed the DBP binding capacity yielding higher 1,25$(OH)_2$D concentrations leading to increased cellular 1,25$(OH)_2$D concentrations.

Hypercalcemia due to vitamin D intoxication is a result of two major actions of vitamin D:

1. Increased absorption of calcium from intestine.
2. Increased calcium resorption from bone via differentiation of osteoclast progenitors into osteoclasts directly and also by an indirect mechanism involving osteoblastic cells.

CLINICAL MANIFESTATIONS

The clinical manifestations of vitamin D toxicity are consequence of high calcium levels. Common manifestations are similar to other hypercalcemic states and include fatigue, generalized weakness, headache, anorexia, polyuria/polydipsia, itching, and dehydration. Gastrointestinal manifestations include constipation, nausea, vomiting, and rarely acute pancreatitis. Central nervous system can be affected and may result in confusion, difficulty in concentration, irritability, drowsiness, and coma. Electrocardiography may show shortened Q–T interval. Ectopic soft tissue calcification can also develop as a result of high calcium and phosphorus product. Risk factors for vitamin D toxicity include extremes of ages, concurrent use of thiazide, impaired renal function, and coexisting disorders such as sarcoidosis and tuberculosis.

DIAGNOSIS OF VITAMIN D TOXICITY

Vitamin D toxicity should be strongly suspected clinically in patients who are being treated with pharmacological dosages of vitamin D. Thorough clinical and drug history is the key in making correct and early diagnosis. Serum 25(OH)D level is the best marker of vitamin D status of an individual. Finding of raised 25(OH)D level (usually >150 ng/mL) and suppressed iPTH in the presence of hypercalcemia confirms the diagnosis of vitamin D toxicity. The iPTH may be raised in presence of coexisting primary hyperparathyroidism or renal failure as illustrated in the above case. $1,25(OH)_2D$ levels are not raised except in setting where overdose of $1,25(OH)_2D$ is responsible for toxicity or in granulomatous disorders due to dysregulated production of $1,25(OH)_2D$. Serum phosphorus levels are either higher side of normal or elevated. Failure to observe elevated 1,25 dihydroxy vitamin D levels in humans with vitamin D toxicity would relegate this metabolite to negligible role in causation of hypercalcemia.

TREATMENT

Vitamin D toxicity needs prompt and aggressive treatment, as it can be life threatening. Treatment modalities are summarized in Table 26.1. Intravenous hydration with normal saline is the first-line treatment of hypercalcemia. Loop diuretics should be used judiciously, as it can exacerbate the existing dehydration. Bisphosphonates and calcitonin comprise additional measures to treat hypercalcemia if hydration alone fails. Glucocorticoids play an important role in treatment of vitamin D toxicity. Mechanisms by which glucocorticoids regulate serum calcium include (a) decrease in synthesis of calcium-binding protein (calbindin-D) and thereby directly inhibiting calcium absorption from gastrointestinal tract, (b) lower 25(OH)D concentrations by altering hepatic vitamin D metabolism, (c) enhance urinary calcium excretion, and (d) inhibit conversion of vitamin D to active form $1,25(OH)_2D$.

Hypercalcemia caused by parent vitamin D overdose can take a long time to normalize due to slow release of vitamin D from fat deposits. Therefore, patient should be followed up regularly with monitoring of serum calcium and 25(OH)D for a period of 1 year. Patient should also be instructed to avoid intake of any calcium or vitamin D supplement.

In our patient, there were at least two risk factors for vitamin D toxicity: old age and chronic kidney disease. The patient was overtreated for vitamin D deficiency that resulted in vitamin D toxicity and associated manifestations. History of intake of such high dose of vitamin D along with raised 25(OH)D

TABLE 26.1: Management of hypercalcemia due to vitamin D toxicity

Therapy	Dose	Mechanism of action
Normal saline	200 mL/h, 100–150 mL/h or according to urine output in elderly and in presence of impaired renal function	Enhances urinary calcium excretion
Loop diuretics Indicated only if aggressive intravenous hydration alone fails to reduce serum calcium	10–20 mg IV 12–24 hourly	Inhibits calcium reabsorption from loop of Henle
Calcitonin	4–8 IU/kg 8–12 hourly SC or IM	Inhibits osteoclast action and bone resorption
Bisphosphonates	Pamidronate: 60–90 mg IV over 2–4 hours, zoledronate: 4 mg IV over 15–30 minutes. Administer half of dose in moderate renal insufficiency	Inhibits osteoclastic bone resorption
Glucocorticoids	Hydrocortisone 200–300 mg IV/day or prednisolone 20–30 mg/day PO	1. Decrease calcium absorption from gut 2. Alters hepatic metabolism of vitamin D to produce more inactive metabolites 3. Enhances urinary calcium excretion 4. Inhibits conversion of vitamin D to active form 1,25(OH)$_2$D

level suggested vitamin D toxicity as likely diagnosis even in the presence of unsuppressed iPTH. The patient was managed promptly for severe hypercalcemia that resulted in decline in serum calcium accompanied by improvement in her sensorium and other clinical manifestations. Glucocorticoids played a significant role in managing hypercalcemia that did not respond to intravenous hydration alone. The raised serum creatinine that could be due to acute kidney injury secondary to dehydration declined with intravenous hydration but did not normalize, indicating pre-existing chronic kidney disease. The patient was readmitted with high serum calcium 1 month after discharge that emphasizes, the need for regular follow-up of cases with vitamin D toxicity as hypercalcemia secondary to vitamin D toxicity is prolonged.

KEY POINTS

- Vitamin D toxicity is most commonly caused by overdose of vitamin D supplements
- Clinical manifestations are secondary to hypercalcemia
- Detailed clinical history is the key to the diagnosis
- Biochemical features include high-serum calcium, high 25(OH)D and suppressed iPTH
- It can be life-threatening if not treated promptly
- Hydration with normal saline is the mainstay of management. Additional measures which are helpful in treating hypercalcemia include judicious use of loop diuretics, calcitonin, bisphosphonates, and glucocorticoids. Hypercalcemia due to parent vitamin D overdose can be prolonged due to slow release of vitamin D from fat deposits. Therefore, regular follow-up with monitoring of serum calcium is needed for at least a year. Prevention includes cautious use of vitamin D supplements and avoidance of parenteral preparation of vitamin D unless there is evidence of malabsorption.

SUGGESTED READINGS

1. Chiricone D, De Santo NG, Cirillo M. Unusual cases of chronic intoxication by vitamin D. J Nephrol. 2003;16(6):917-21.
2. Jones G. Pharmacokinetics of vitamin D toxicity. Am J Clin Nutr. 2008;88(2):582S-6S.
3. Klontz KC, Acheson DW. Dietary supplement-induced vitamin D intoxication. N Engl J Med. 2007;357(3):308-9.
4. Koutkia P, Chen TC, Holick MF. Vitamin D intoxication associated with an over-the-counter supplement. N Engl J Med. 2001;345(1):66-7.
5. Leu JP, Weiner A, Barzel US. Vitamin D toxicity: caveat emptor. Endocr Pract. 2008;14(9):1188-90.
6. Mithal A, Wahl DA, Bonjour JP, et al. Global vitamin D status and determinants of hypovitaminosis D. Osteoporos Int. 2009;20(11):1807-20.

CHAPTER

27

Diabetes Mellitus in Hypopituitarism

Narasimha KR Setty, Surekha B Shetty

CASE PRESENTATION

A 57-year-old female with a known history of "hypertension" for the last 10 years was diagnosed to have type 2 diabetes mellitus 6 months ago. She presented with a history of tiredness and easy fatigability for past few months. She is very lethargic and finds it difficult to carry out daily routine activities. Patient denies any previous history of cardiopulmonary disease, hepatic disease, or renal disease. No history of fever, weight gain/loss, or diarrhea was reported. No symptoms of hypoglycemia were reported.

Past medical history: Patient has a history of secondary amenorrhea since age of 22 years following completion of her second pregnancy. It was a twin pregnancy and was uneventful until delivery. However, both newborn babies died within few days after delivery. There was no history of pre/postpartum hemorrhage or hypotension requiring treatment. The amenorrhea was not evaluated or treated. Patient was otherwise asymptomatic till recently. Review of medical records revealed thyroid profile reports with low serum thyroxine and triiodothyronine with "normal" thyroid-stimulating hormone (TSH) for the last 10 years.

Physical examination: Patient was moderately built and nourished, with height of 154 cm, weight of 65 kg, and body mass index (BMI) of 27.4.

Heart rate was 60 per minute, and blood pressure was 130/80 mmHg with no postural drop. Systemic examination was normal. Her neurologic examination was unremarkable.

LABORATORY INVESTIGATIONS

- Hemoglobin, 11.9 g/dL (normal: 12–14.5 g/dL]; white blood cell (WBC) count 6,600/cum
- Total cholesterol, 286 mg/dL; triglycerides, 327 mg/dL

- Blood urea, 20 mg/dL; serum creatinine, 1.1 mg/dL
- Serum sodium, 137 mEq/L; serum potassium, 3.69 mEq/L; serum chloride, 96 mEq/L
- Fasting blood glucose: 166 mg/dL (normal: 70–99 mg/dL)
- 2 Hours postprandial glucose: 286 mg/dL (normal: <140 mg/dL)
- Glycosylated hemoglobin (HbA1c): 8.1%
- T3: 0.633 nmol/L (normal: 1.3–3.10 nmol/L)
- T4: 28 nmol/L (normal: 66–174 nmol/L)
- Thyroid-stimulating hormone (TSH): 3.36 µIU/mL (normal: 0.27–4.2 µIU/mL)
- Free T3: 3.58 pmol/L (normal: 3.1-6.8 pmol/L)
- Free T4: 3.33 pmol/L (normal: 12–22 pmol/L)
- Luteinizing hormone (LH)/follicle-stimulating hormone (FSH): 0.35 mIU/mL
- Serum prolactin: 0.41 ng/mL (normal: 4.8–23.2)
- Fasting growth hormone (GH): 0.06 ng/mL
- Basal plasma cortisol: 4.66 µg/dL (normal: 7–20 µg/dL)
- Plasma cortisol after Synacthen* stimulation: 11.91 µg/dL.

IMAGING STUDIES

- Magnetic resonance imaging (MRI) brain: Empty sella. Posterior pituitary hyperintensity not visualized (Figs 27.1 and 27.2).

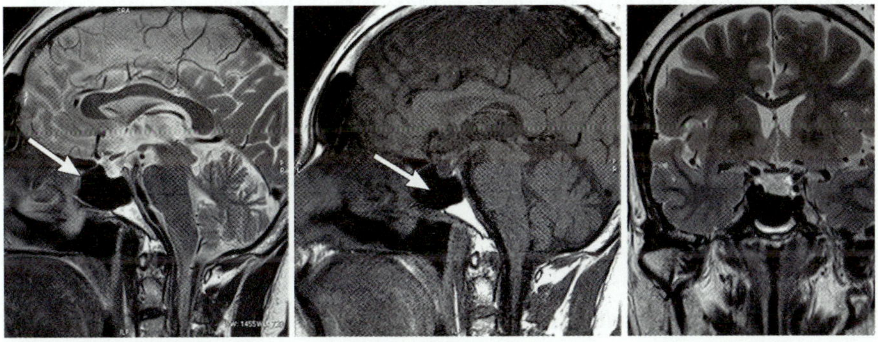

Figure 27.1: Sagittal T2-, T1-, and coronal T2-weighted images of pituitary sella, demonstrating empty sella

**Synacthen (Tetracosactrin):* Synthetic preparation of first 24 amino acids of natural adrenocorticotropic hormone (ACTH).

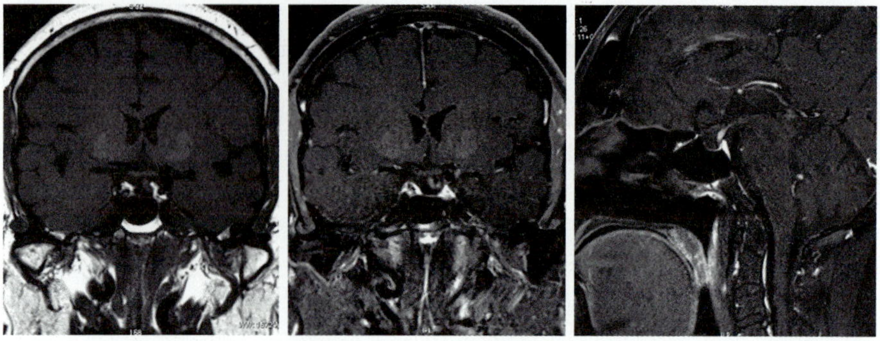

Figure 27.2: Noncontrast coronal T1 with postcontrast coronal and sagittal T1-weighted images of the pituitary sella, demonstrating empty sella

DIAGNOSIS

- Type 2 diabetes mellitus: Uncontrolled
- Dyslipidemia-Fredrickson type IIb
- Postpartum pan-hypopituitarism.

TREATMENT

Patient was placed on medical nutrition therapy with advice to lose 5–7% weight and asked to return for follow-up in 12 weeks. She received glucocorticoid and thyroid hormone replacement therapy. A bone density study was ordered and estrogen replacement therapy discussed and a decision was made not to replace. Bone health treatment would be decided following completion of bone densitometry study. Repeat hormonal studies were ordered in 4 weeks following initiation of therapy.

We anticipate improvement in her anemia and glycemic control. Upon return in 12 weeks, improvement in glycemic control was noticed.

DISCUSSION

Sheehan's syndrome refers to state of hypopituitarism consequent to necrosis of the pituitary gland occurring due to severe postpartum hemorrhage/ hypotension. Enlargement of pituitary gland, small sellar size, disseminated intravascular coagulation, and autoimmunity during pregnancy may play a role in its pathogenesis. The extent of anterior pituitary dysfunction has varied in different series. At least 75% of the anterior pituitary must be destroyed before clinical manifestations become evident. The order of diminished trophic hormone reserve function related to pituitary dysfunction usually is as follows: GH > FSH > LH > TSH > ACTH. However, this is not necessary order in many patients. Prolactin levels fall with resultant failure of lactation.

An epidemiological study from the Kashmir valley estimated the prevalence to be about 3% in women above 20 years of age. Sheehan's syndrome can present in the postpartum period with lactation failure or after many months to years following the delivery. In many affected women, anterior pituitary dysfunction is not diagnosed for many years.

Characteristic manifestations include failure to lactate, amenorrhea, weakness, dry skin, hypopigmentation, and anemia. Uncommonly, it can present acutely with circulatory collapse, severe hyponatremia, hypoglycemia, or psychosis. In elderly, the presentation is often nonspecific with symptoms such as lethargy, pallor, falls, urinary incontinence, and confusion. Hence, high index of suspicion is needed for diagnosis of this situation.

The role of pituitary in glucose homeostasis was first demonstrated by Houssay and Biasotti in 1931, when they showed that the post-pancreatectomy diabetes in experimental dogs could be alleviated by removal of anterior pituitary (Houssay phenomenon). Conversely, the development of diabetes was reported in dogs following prolonged administration of anterior pituitary extracts (Young 1937).

The Houssay phenomenon in humans would follow injury to anterior pituitary in patients with diabetes mellitus. It manifests as increase in sensitivity to both endogenous and exogenous insulin and propensity to hypoglycemia. As a corollary, it was assumed that it should be unusual to find patients with pre-existing hypopituitarism developing diabetes mellitus. This concept must be revisited in the context of increasing obesity/adiposity that brings with its significant insulin resistance. Indeed both the KIMS (*Pfizer—formerly Kabi, international metabolic study database*) and HypoCCS (*hypopituitarism control and complications study*) yielded increased prevalence of impaired glucose tolerance and diabetes in adult-onset GH deficiency patients even before GH replacement. In both instances, it was related to adverse body composition. Much of the diabetogenic influence of pituitary has been ascribed to GH. The now abandoned practice of hypophysectomy to treat diabetic retinopathy was rooted in this notion.

Literature is peppered with cases reports that seem to foster the notion that diabetes must be highly uncommon in a state of pre-existing hypopituitarism, and therefore, worthy of reporting. Our case highlights the perils of such dogmatic view. If hypopituitarism was to evolve in an established patient with diabetes mellitus, pituitary insufficiency must be excluded after any other possible etiology has been excluded as cause for increased frequency and severity of hypoglycemia.

In a patient with diabetes and concurrent hypopituitarism, there is no contraindication to use of currently available antihyperglycemic therapies. However, attention must be paid to avoid overzealous hormone replacement that could potentially adversely impact body composition, and insulin sensitivity.

KEY POINTS

- Clinical features of hypopituitarism are often subtle and years may pass before the diagnosis is made
- History of postpartum hemorrhage, failure to lactate, and amenorrhea are important clues to the diagnosis. Early diagnosis and appropriate treatment are necessary to reduce the morbidity and mortality in these patients
- Occurrence of diabetes in a patient with pre-existing hypopituitarism is no longer a rare phenomenon
- Glucocorticoid deficiency and hypothyroidism do not offer protection against diabetes mellitus and that insulin resistance, often encountered in obesity, is sufficient to override any such perceived protection.

SUGGESTED READINGS

1. Abs R, Mattsson AF, Thunander M, et al. Prevalence of diabetes mellitus in 6050 hypopituitary patients with adult-onset GH deficiency before GH replacement: a KIMS analysis. Eur J Endocrinol. 2013;168:297-305.
2. Attanasio AF, Jung H, Mo D, et al. Prevalence and incidence of diabetes mellitus in adult patients on growth hormone replacement for growth hormone deficiency. A surveillance database analysis. J Clin Endocrinol Metab. 2011;96:2255-61.
3. Grunberg A, Blair JL. Hypopituitarism with consecutive development of diabetes mellitus. Br Med J. 1957; August 24:439-41.
4. Houssay BA, Biasotti A. The hypophysis, carbohydrate mechanism and diabetes. Endocrinology. 1931;15:511-23.
5. Lufi R, Olivecrona H, Ikkos D, et al. Hypophysectomy in man. Further experiences in sever diabetes mellitus. Br Med J. 1955;2:752-6.
6. Young FC. The pancreotropic action of anterior pituitary extracts. J Physiol. 1937;91:352-64.
7. Zargar AH, Singh B, Laway BA, et al. Epidemiologic aspects of postpartum pituitary hypofunction (Sheehan's syndrome). Fertil Steril. 2005;84:523-8.

Index

Page numbers followed by *f* refer to figure and *t* refer to table.

A

E

F

G

H

I

J

K

L

M

N

O

P

R

S

T

U

V

W

Z